GERONTOLOGY IN HIGHER EDUCATION:

Perspectives and Issues

Editors:

**Mildred M. Seltzer
Harvey Sterns
Tom Hickey**

**Papers from the 1977 Meeting of the
Association for Gerontology in Higher Education**

Wadsworth Publishing Company, Inc. Belmont, California

Gerontology Editor: Stephen D. Rutter
Production Editor: Anne D. Kelly
Designer: Cynthia A. Bassett

Printed in the United States of America
1 2 3 4 5 6 7 8 9 10—82 81 80 79 78

Library of Congress Cataloging in Publication Data

Main entry under title:

Gerontology today in higher education.

    Papers selected from the proceedings of the Association's annual meeting.
    1.   Gerontology—Study and teaching (Higher)—United
States—Congresses.   I.   Seltzer, Mildred M., date
II.   Sterns, Harvey.   III.   Hickey, Tom, 1939—
IV. Association for Gerontology in Higher Education.
HQ1061.G42   362.6'042'071173   77-28079
ISBN 0-534-00582-9

CONTENTS

INTRODUCTION

This commentary is a collection of papers on gerontology and higher education. For the most part, these papers were selected from invited presentations at the 1977 annual meeting of the Association for Gerontology in Higher Education. This volume represents both the selected proceedings of this annual meeting and an experimental effort towards the eventual publication of an annual monograph or review of Aging and Higher Education.

While it is true that meetings, conferences, and proceedings in the past have focused on gerontology in higher education, the 1977 AGHE annual meeting provided evidence that a transition has been taking place. In the past we just talked about the need for programs and funding policies, and we mutually shared curriculum ideas and program models. But the present transition period reflects our movement beyond mere sharing-and-telling. We are now making somewhat structured attempts to define the future on a different conceptual level of organization. Although structure here might imply some rigidity of boundaries, there is always room for continued innovation. In the development of gerontology for higher education we have reached a point where basic principles and frameworks must be codified to prevent unnecessarily repeating our past.

The obvious variation in priorities expressed in these papers as well as their uneven quality reflects our current state. There are multiple perspectives of gerontology in higher education, and these perspectives vary significantly in the degree to which they are defined and developed. The papers and commentaries also reflect the wide range in program focus from community college to graduate university, and from single or topical programs to multidisciplinary and consortia activities. Moreover, these perspectives vary significantly in the degree to which they are defined and developed. This volume therefore reflects our current status—admittedly unrefined in many areas.

In preparing this volume, the editors at first considered a traditional academic approach of qualitatively selecting, distilling, and editing the "major" papers. However, it became apparent to us that the current state-of-the-field—at least many of the important emerging areas of the field—is more evident in the informal dialogues and commentaries. The selection of papers and commentaries reflects the broad issues with which we are and have been concerned: teaching, program administration, research development, and the community relationship of our educational programs. Levels of development in these areas are quite variable, and the commentaries suggest this in their occasional redundancy and uneven quality. The major papers in this volume provide a good overview of the key issues facing gerontology in higher education today. The commentary papers represent the broader and more wide-ranging thinking about how we will deal with these issues in the future. The communication of these ideas and issues to gerontologists nation-wide should carry us an important step forward in the development of effective educational strategies for gerontology.

In an era of many national organizations, associational meetings, workshops, journals and other organized professional media, this book is a useful and important perspective to share, as it represents a cross-section of higher education's programs in gerontology. In a presidential address to the 1977 annual meeting, Tom Hickey noted that gerontology was beginning an important third stage in its development. The first stage was represented by unstructured acquisitiveness or interest in aging from various sectors. The next period—emerging most visibly after the passage of the Older Americans Act in the mid 1960s—was characterized by the establishment of organized constituencies in the policy, research, education, and service areas. In the emerging third stage, the constituencies are learning the tensions of working together, a difficult challenge in the face of limited resources. Thus, by sharing the current status of gerontology in higher education we are attempting to stimulate further the effective and nonduplicative development of educational programs, as well as to increase the value and relevance of the relationship between education and society's needs as expressed through the other constituencies.

The Association for Gerontology in Higher Education fulfills an important constituency role on behalf of colleges and universities. It is both an educational and an institutional role that neither institution nor faculty can assume effectively on an individual basis, and it is one that cannot be ignored. Moreover, the institutional structure of AGHE further protects our academic freedom in research and instruction. As individual faculty members and/or as members of our professional groups—especially the Gerontological Society—we can continue to speak out on behalf of policy, research, and related instructional issues regardless of institutional positions. This is important to ensure continued creative growth in the future.

In order to put this selection of papers and commentaries into a somewhat historical context—our "roots" so to speak—we have included an outline summary of the Association for Gerontology in Higher Education as Part One. This brief history focuses on the purposes that initially drew gerontology educators together, the eventual development of the Association and its mission, and its subsequent activities over the past five years.

PART ONE
HISTORY AND BACKGROUND

Association for Gerontology in Higher Education—A Brief History

Tom Hickey
University of Michigan

I. The Association for Gerontology in Higher Education began as the Ad Hoc Committee on the Development of Gerontology Resources at Brandeis University in May, 1972.

This ad hoc committee was initially formed to mobilize gerontology resources to adequately respond to the Administration on Aging's proposal for the establishment of regional gerontology centers. Members of the committee emerged from a long-standing informal group of educators—typically Training Program Directors (AoA, Titles IV and V)—that was convened twice annually by AoA to discuss gerontological education.

II. At a second meeting (August, 1972), the ad hoc committee broadened its purpose to consider the general question of how best to mobilize universities to respond to the new demands of public policy regarding training and research to provide public services for the elderly. Subcommittees were formed to further define and delineate this purpose, and members of the committee were asked to assess the state of gerontological research and training within their (HEW) region. These tasks were addressed with great urgency, given the political context at that time when the federal decision-making systems were functioning with little professional input or peer review.

Robert Binstock (Brandeis University) chaired this group; Mary Wylie (University of Wisconsin) directed preparation of the resource document;

Merrill Elias (University of West Virginia) served as recorder-secretary; and Frances Scott (University of Oregon) also served on this committee.

Other institutions sent representatives, and the following individuals were subsequently elected to serve as HEW Regional Reporters:

Region 1: Frank Carter (New England Center for Continuing Education)
Region 2: Walter Beattie (Syracuse University)
Region 3: Tom Hickey (Pennsylvania State University)
Region 4: Albert Wilson (University of Southern Florida)
Region 5: Wayne Vasey (University of Michigan)
Region 6: Hiram Friedsam (North Texas State University)
Region 7: Warren Peterson (University of Missouri, Kansas City)
Region 8: Melvin White (University of Utah)
Region 9: Ruth Weg (University of Southern California)

III. Two months later, in October of 1972, the ad hoc committee reconvened at Newport Beach, California, to consider and make recommendations about the following issues:

    A. A seven-part definition of Multidisciplinary Centers of Gerontology (Congressional Record, October 4, 1972):

        1. "Recruit and train personnel at the professional and subprofessional levels."

        2. "Conduct basic and applied research on work, leisure, and education of older people, living arrangements of older people, social services for older people, the economics of aging, and other related areas."

        3. "Provide consultation to public and voluntary organizations with respect to the needs of older people and in planning and developing services for them."

        4. "Serve as a repository of information and knowledge with respect to the areas for which it conducts basic and applied research."

        5. "Stimulate the incorporation of information on aging into the teaching of biological, behavioral, and social sciences at colleges or universities."

        6. "Help to develop training programs on aging in schools of social work, public health, health care administration, education, and in other such schools at colleges and universities."

        7. "Create opportunities for innovative, multidisciplinary efforts in teaching, research, and demonstration projects with respect to aging."

    B. Issues raised by the concept of regional centers vis-à-vis the proper role, structure, and function of universities to mobilize resources (Beattie):

        1. Critical question: What is the best way in which to mobilize the resources of institutions of higher learning so that they may respond in an effective manner to the new demands of public

policy for the training of staff and research relative to the provision of services for the elderly? (How do universities relate to each other and to the government in order to respond to new demands of public policy?)

2. Facts:
   a. Regions vary, not only in geographic diversity, but also in resources and needs. Institutions of higher learning vary greatly according to: auspices—public and private; location—urban, suburban, and rural; tradition—some emphasize research and training while others emphasize community technical assistance and continuing community education; and structures—through which they achieve these objectives.
   b. The structure of institutions of higher learning varies; therefore, their functions vary.

3. Assumptions:
   a. We are dealing with diversity. No single model will be sufficient for all institutions of higher learning and all areas of the country.
   b. Structure, function, and objectives of the government are not necessarily isomorphic with the structure, function, and objectives of institutions of higher learning.
   c. Diversity is a strength of institutions of higher learning. It provides the capability to respond to a variety of demands of government and public policy, when those demands are consistent with its structure, function, and objectives.

4. The objectives and functions of higher education (it should be noted that they include and go beyond the goals outlined by Title V legislation):
   a. Planning and evaluation of educational resources
   b. Sharing of scarce resources
   c. Consulting and assisting in the development of criteria for review with the objective of insuring quality of function
   d. Facilitating relationships between institutions of higher learning and various levels of government, i.e., serving as negotiator between government and the institution
   e. Participating in advanced planning for the development of long- and short-term educational and training resources
   f. Participating in policy-making decisions with regard to education and training in gerontology
   g. Serving as a broker between resources in a region and the government. Institutions may properly serve as a broker in terms of communication and coordination, but they should not intervene in the awarding of federal resources.

h. Integrating the efforts of multiple federal agencies
5. Conclusions:
   a. The assumptions and functions outlined above indicate the necessity of multiple institutions with diverse functions since few institutions have the resources to engage in all functions.
   b. There are a diverse number of relationships that can be formed between institutions of higher education and the government.
6. Structure:
   a. A center can take many forms. It may refer to one or many institutions. These institutions may engage in activities that are national in scope or they may involve particular regions or states.
   b. A center would be expected to draw upon identified resources in the zone in which it functions.
      1) There may be one campus or many campuses.
      2) These campuses and their activities may be interrelated and mutually reinforcing.
7. At this point, it is premature and inappropriate to make specific recommendations with regard to structure.
C. The potential usefulness of a national association of institutions of higher learning that would serve to coordinate activities with regard to the mobilization of gerontology resources (Vasey):
   1. Organization of local, state, and regional associations may more properly precede the development of a national association.
   2. There are definite local, state, and regional training needs which must be met, and all institutions of higher education within these localities, states, and regions must be given an opportunity to participate in meeting these needs. A national association could help define the role of centers of gerontology in institutions of higher learning in meeting these needs in an effective and appropriate manner.
   3. A national association should have as one of its purposes advocacy of a peer review system for research and for training and development grants submitted to the Administration on Aging and other federal agencies. This means that a national association could sustain the concept of accountability for maintenance of educational standards with all institutions within a region given the opportunity to participate in a peer review system.
   4. The Gerontological Society should be requested to serve as a convener of representatives of institutions of higher education in gerontology to consider the future, form, and structure of a national organization.

D. The future steps in the direction of improving the lines of communication between institutions of higher learning and the government (Eli Cohen, University of Pennsylvania):
    1. A peer review system should be instigated with the development of study sections within the AoA. It should be instigated for both training and research grants, and it should be organized on national and regional levels. The gerontological expertise within universities should be utilized in such peer review.
    2. Increased effort on the part of the academic community is necessary in order to increase student involvement in the articulation, planning, and evaluation of training and training needs. Evaluation of training and training needs may be achieved through:
        a. Internships with the federal government and other agencies
        b. Work study programs with the federal government and other agencies
E. The conclusions and recommendations reached by the three subcommittees were unanimously endorsed by the ad hoc committee with the following stipulations:
    1. Further discussions should be conducted with regard to the exact wording.
    2. Conclusions and recommendations are not to be viewed as binding decisions; rather, they are objectives, principles, and guidelines that will provide direction for the next meeting.
F. At the conclusion of this meeting, the ad hoc committee agreed to meet in January of 1973; and the following changes were made in the executive committee in the interests of sharing the significant time and resource involvement of the executive committee members and their respective universities to date: Walter Beattie replaced Robert Binstock; Leonard Gottesman (Philadelphia Geriatric Center) replaced Mary Wylie; Bernice Neugarten replaced Frances Scott; Merrill Elias (now Syracuse University) remained for continuity.

IV. On January 25–26, 1973, the ad hoc committee met in Washington, D.C., to deal with three issues:
A. The preparation and submission of a written set of recommendations to the federal government regarding the mobilization of training resources for manpower needs
B. The preparation of a resource document
C. The structure of organizational continuity to assure that following the dissolution of the ad hoc committee, its recommendations would continue to be conveyed in a personalized, dynamic, and forceful manner

In addition, the committee invited various federal representatives and officials to address its meeting informally. These included Dr. Arthur Flemming (Special Advisor to President Nixon), Dr. Marvin Taves (Administration on Aging), and William Oriol (Senate Committee on Aging).

This meeting resulted in a consensus that some form of continuity of the committee was vital to facilitate interinstitutional communication regarding institutional program development. It was agreed that there was no organized forum to accomplish this goal—especially from the *institutional* perspective of higher education programs in aging. Although a committee or structured organization should relate to, work with, or otherwise affiliate formally with the Gerontological Society, it was agreed to keep communications open informally for the present time via interface with the Education Committee of the Society.

A new executive committee was elected to direct their attention to the structure of a continuing organization and to make recommendations to the other ad hoc committee members, Wayne Vasey, Chair; Tom Hickey, Secretary; Ruth Weg, Structure of Membership; John O'Brien (Portland State University), Organizational Structure; Walter Beattie, Fiscal Strategy; and Robert Binstock, *ex officio* for the purpose of concluding contracted reports to AoA related to the first two issues on this agenda.

V. On April 9–10, 1973, the Ad Hoc Committee on the Development of Gerontology Resources met again in Washington. This meeting focused on two issues:

    A. The impending crisis for training and education funds for aging

    B. The continuity of the committee in view of the emerging need for strong constituencies to counteract the funding crisis

Prior to and during this meeting, there was much substantive discussion between the executive committee and various representatives of the federal government and Congress regarding major policy, fiscal, and structural changes—dictated largely by the Office of Management and the Budget—which would lead to the overall weakening of the field, and the specific dissolution of many gerontology programs in institutions of higher education. Thus, much of the meeting was devoted to the development of strategies for countering this impending crisis. For the most part, these strategies were based substantively on the 1971 White House Conference on Aging reports, and tactically on the communication of relevant information about this educational field to the appropriate elected and appointed officials.

In the course of this meeting the current name—Association for Gerontology in Higher Education (AGHE)—was selected on the basis of earlier recommendations by Bernice Neugarten and a motion by Erdman Palmore (Duke University).

In the interests of strengthening the professional constituency in time of crisis, the Association agreed to formally affiliate with the Gerontological Society and charged its Executive Committee to continue to study structural issues as well as the major priority of federal policy in regard to training and education. Although many structural issues were discussed at this meeting, the federal policy issue and the appropriate substantive response consumed the greater part of the agenda.

VI. During the summer and fall of 1973, members of the Executive Committee continued to be active on behalf of the Association in areas related to policy and regularly reported back to the member institutions (now numbering 31) and their representatives.

At its annual meeting in Miami Beach (November, 1973), the Council of the Gerontological Society voted for an affiliation with AGHE which would:

A. Have a liaison structure between the Council of the Gerontological Society and the Executive Committee of AGHE
B. Maintain autonomous decision-making and action-taking authority
C. Seek collaborative and mutually beneficial cooperative relationships with the Gerontological Society

Affiliation is subject to evaluation and review after three years by both Associations.

VII. On February 28, 1974, representatives of member institutions of AGHE met in Chicago to review the policy and structure issues.

A series of activities and subsequent recommendations in the policy area were discussed, and the emergence of evidence of success at the Washington level were noted and appreciated by the membership.

The following structural issues were considered:

A. Discussion and tentative agreements to first drafts of Articles of Incorporation and Bylaws
B. Discussion of tax-exempt and lobbying-status problems, resolving to have AGHE reflect a (nonlobbying) 501 (c) (3) tax status
C. Designation of Attorney Richard Verville of Washington, D.C., as registered agent. There was much subsequent discussion of using his office as a central office, and contracting with him (subject to AGHE's fiscal affluence) for additional services vis-à-vis monitoring federal legislation related to AGHE purposes and the interests of its institutional members.
D. Agreement to institutional membership only
E. Decision for elected officers to serve until the first official annual meeting to be held after incorporation: Walter Beattie, President; Martin Loeb (University of Wisconsin), President-elect; Mildred Seltzer (Miami University), Secretary; John O'Brien, Treasurer; and Wayne Vasey, Past-president

VIII. A general informational meeting of the Association was held in Ann Arbor, Michigan, in August, 1974, in conjunction with an educational program of special interest to AGHE members, convened by Wayne Vasey and the Institute of Gerontology.

The Executive Committee of AGHE met during the following month in Washington to pursue policy issues with federal officials—with continuing evidence of success as determined by renewed funding of many member programs as well as changes in federal policy directions.

AGHE held a general meeting of its membership on October 31, in conjunction with the annual meeting of the Gerontological Society in Portland, Oregon.

   A. The legal status of the Association for Gerontology in Higher Education, Inc., was noted.
   B. Final organizational details were resolved.
   C. The first annual meeting of the incorporated Association was scheduled.
   D. A general report regarding public policy positions of the Association was made to the membership.

IX. The first annual meeting of the Association was held in Madison, Wisconsin, on April 6–8, 1975. With most organizational details accomplished, this successful meeting focused on substantive issues of interest to the general membership; the AGHE purpose of facilitating interinstitutional communication and program development was the primary focus. Attendance exceeded 100 people, many of whom were prospective new members. In addition, representatives of Congress and many different federal agencies attended and participated in the formal program.

The following members were elected to office: Tom Hickey, President-elect; Mildred Seltzer, Secretary; David Peterson (University of Nebraska), Treasurer; Ann Hudis (Hunter College) and Ira Ehrlich (St. Louis University), Members-at-large.

X. During 1975, the following major activities took place:

   A. The development of a new Resource Directory of Education Programs in Gerontology was undertaken under contract with the AoA.
   B. A technical assistance contract with the Veterans Administration was established for the purpose of developing educational and research programs related both to VA and AGHE member institution goals.
   C. The Proceedings of the Madison meeting were published and distributed.
   D. The affiliation status with the Gerontological Society was reaffirmed with the delineation of specific activities and program goals.
   E. The second annual meeting of the Association was scheduled for March 3–5, 1976, in Chevy Chase, Maryland, with the program to include a special hearing on education and other aging related issues by the House of Representatives Select Committee on Aging.
   F. A central office was established within the Gerontological Society's Washington offices.
   G. Program goals and the necessary subcommittee structures were set in place by the President-elect for 1976–77, in order to facilitate both an increasing momentum and continuity, as well as to minimize organizational details at the second annual meeting (with the exception of routine and typical "tidying-up" of the Bylaws).

XI. The second annual meeting of the Association for Gerontology in Higher Education was held in Chevy Chase, Maryland, on March 3–5, 1976. The meeting carried a dual focus:
   A. Substantive issues of interest for gerontological program development in institutions of higher education.
   B. Communication with the federal legislative process.
A highlight of the meeting was a public hearing at the Capitol conducted by the House Select Subcommittee on Aging. Officers of the Association presented formal testimony, and over 100 meeting participants attended.

The following members were elected to office: Hiram Friedsam, President-elect; Erdman Palmore (Duke University), Secretary; and Donald Spence (University of Rhode Island), Member-at-large.

XII. During the remainder of 1976 a number of activities were initiated to more fully operationalize the objectives of the Association as well as many of the preceding recommendations contained in this history.
   A. The Public Policy committee continued its activities on behalf of AGHE. These included more frequent communication with the federal legislative process, collaborative policy activities with the Gerontological Society, legislative staff consultations, presentation of testimony to various public Hearings of the Legislative and Executive branches of the federal government, and activities on state and local levels. A limited form of peer review of AoA training and education proposals continued for the second year.
   B. The flow of communications back to the membership increased with routine policy and informational bulletins, and with quarterly newsletters containing program guides and other useful information. Active participation by the membership in local and regional policy forums and increased interinstitutional communications resulted from these bulletins and newsletters.
   C. A *National Directory of Educational Programs in Gerontology* (containing approximately 1,200 entries) was published in 1976.
   D. In affiliation with the Gerontological Society, the Association cosponsored a Summer Institute for Educators and Researchers.
   E. The financial status of the Association continued to stabilize and improve, with all membership and financial activities managed from the central office in Washington, D.C.
   F. Annual meeting sites were projected for 3 years ahead:
   1977: Tucson, February 23–25
   1978: Dallas, March 8–10
   1979: Washington, D.C.
   G. A symposium on Education for Allied Health Professions was conducted at the Gerontological Society's annual meeting in New York (October 13–17, 1976) in conjunction with the Society's Clinical Medicine Section.

H. The ad hoc committee for long-range planning formalized a Concept and Mission Statement which was endorsed by the Executive Committee at their June meeting at Penn State. This led to the development of a project proposal in collaboration with the Gerontological Society to lay the groundwork for educational program guidelines—a continuing recommendation in the preceding pages of this history.

PART TWO
MAJOR ISSUES

Section One

Major Issues:
Current Perspectives

This section contains the presentations of those dealing with general and broad perspectives of education in gerontology. The authors of these papers discuss what they consider the major issues confronting people engaged in teaching and research about aging. They review the present and anticipate future issues.

An Overview of Gerontology Education

David A. Peterson
University of Nebraska

One of the responsibilities which American institutions of higher education have accepted during the past century is the application of knowledge and methods from the various disciplines to the problems which confront society. Although not the sole purpose of higher education, this operational stance has encouraged many colleges, community colleges, and universities to initiate teaching, research, and community service activities which are relevant to the expressed and assumed needs of older people in contemporary society. This gerontologically related activity has taken many forms, but a major portion of it has been in the area of instruction designed to prepare personnel for employment in agencies and institutions which provide services to older people.

Donahue (1963), Hickey (1976), and Orbach (1976) have provided reviews of the development of these activities. Rather than attempting to supplement their commentaries, the purpose of this paper is to describe the contemporary situation in a manner which will be of use to faculty and administrators interested in developing gerontology education and to raise a number of issues which should be considered in such an undertaking. It is not anticipated that all of the issues will be resolved in this paper, but rather that by focusing attention on them, those planning and developing gerontology education may be in a better position to make the basic decisions which will affect the long-term outcomes of the programs.

After several years of discussions at professional meetings and conferences, it appears that most gerontology educators would agree that gerontology is an interdisciplinary study of the process of aging. Content is drawn from several of the natural and social sciences so that the psychological, physical, and social processes of development in the later stages of life are emphasized. Although gerontology indicates the *study* of later life, closely associated is the *field of service* to older people which often stresses social concern, political advocacy, and intemperate gushiness. It is difficult to separate these elements, and gerontology instructors frequently find themselves involved in the current problems and programs which were designed to assist vulnerable older people. Thus, at the start, we should be aware that we are not dealing only with an area of social or biological science, but that aspects of public policy, human service, and humanistic ideology are also frequently interwoven with the more traditional content.

Development of Interest in Older People

The growth of public interest in and concern for older people in the U.S. somewhat preceded the development of activities within institutions of higher education designed to assist this vulnerable group. However, recent developments both within higher education and in the larger society have generated an awareness by both faculty and administrators of this academic and professional area.

The rapid increase in the size and proportion of the older population has doubtless been a significant impetus to elevating the level of concern for this population. This has been supplemented by a general increase in social consciousness which led to the creation of the Great Society programs of the 1960s and by the realization that the future growth of the older population will affect the economic, social, and political bases on which our society rests.

The result has been a substantial growth in human service programs which are designed to alleviate the difficulties of disadvantaged groups. Federal financing of programs for the retarded, physically handicapped, mentally ill, unemployed, and aged has expanded not only the services available, but also the employment opportunities for professionals and paraprofessionals whose interests and skills are relevant to these populations.

These job opportunities have expanded at the time when some of the more traditional markets have begun to contract. This has caused college students and their faculty advisors to examine more closely and seriously the professional opportunities which the human services present. Because of the large number of older persons, their political activism, and the coverage which they were being provided in the media, new courses and programs to prepare persons to work in the area of aging have been established over the past ten years.

At the same time, researchers and concerned practitioners were generating increasing amounts of data which could be used in better understanding and serving older clients. As this body of knowledge grew and authors began to present it in a systematic manner, the materials for use in these instructional programs gained wide acceptance by faculty members desiring to include some information about aging in the courses which they were teaching or intended to develop.

Federal government agencies such as the Administration on Aging and the National Institutes of Health encouraged this development by providing financial aid to students interested in a career in the area of aging and by supplying funds for faculty salaries and operational costs. This federal aid has become an amount which is of substantial interest to educational institutions that have experienced a reduction in federal funding or have not previously had the opportunity to compete for outside support. Thus, many institutions of higher education have initiated research, education, and public service projects in the area of aging.

Undergraduate and graduate course work in gerontology has shown a substantial increase in the last five years. In 1976, the AGHE survey of higher education done by the staff of the University of Wisconsin identified 1,275 educational institutions involved in aging-related activity. The distribution of these programs was great, with each state having some activity but no state comprising more than 8 percent of the total. Junior and community colleges made up 33 percent of this activity; four-year colleges comprised 29 percent; and universities made up 27 percent. At least 600 of the institutions responding to the survey had at least one credit course in gerontology and over 400 had two or more courses. Two hundred and sixty institutions had some kind of a program of study in gerontology. These programs were described in various ways: 51 institutions had a major in gerontology; 10 had a minor; 33 had some content in gerontology; 31 had a concentration; 24 had a sequence; and 29 had some other designation which described the type of program which was available.

It should be expected that the future will hold continued development of gerontology instruction. Two hundred and ninety of the institutions indicated that they expect to develop more courses in the area; 172 anticipate the development of a program of study leading to a credential in gerontology; and 21 expect to develop a gerontology center.

These developments are exciting and important. Yet they also raise many issues in regard to the purposes, outcomes, and quality of the activities which are being undertaken. Up to this time, most persons concerned with gerontology education have assumed that the major issue for the field was how to encourage the development of more instruction in the area. Recently, however, it is possible to detect a change in this position. More and more faculty and administrators are beginning to ask whether there are not other questions which also need to be raised. Questions such as what levels of instruction should receive priority in development? What content should be emphasized? And what purposes should be encouraged? There certainly is a need for the expansion of gerontology education, but it is evident that additional planning and evaluation will be required if we are to avoid extreme competition, overlap, and confusion.

Definition of Gerontology Education

Before moving along too far, it is important to define the topic that is being dealt with. Gerontology education is the study of the area of aging at the post-secondary level. It often involves traditional course work within a collegiate setting, but other formats such as workshops and conferences are also popular. It should be distinguished from the education of older people, which is also a growing area of interest, but which typically focuses on providing retirees non-credit instruction in coping skills or in continuing their personal or intellectual development in the later years.

Gerontology education can normally be divided into two somewhat separate classifications: (1) preservice education, which generally is undertaken during the earlier stages of life and is meant as preparation for a professional role or to assist in intellectual development; and (2) continuing education, which typically is provided after the formal stages of education are completed and which is likely to be of use to the individual in maintaining and improving professional and personal skills.

The continuing education of professionals in the field of aging has become a very large activity. There are currently dozens of conferences, workshops, and institutes which are available to those who wish to participate in them. However, these activities tend to be somewhat peripheral to our major interest. Consequently, a focus on the preservice education seems more appropriate.

Preservice education can be undertaken in two contexts. These involve (1) the preparation of professionals and paraprofessionals for work in research, education, administration, or delivery of services relevant to the target population, and (2) the education of undergraduate and graduate students in order to transmit an understanding of the process of aging and the roles older people play in contemporary society without regard to the utilization of this knowledge in a professional capacity. In other words, the gerontology education may be oriented toward professional practice or personal understanding—the old dichotomy of vocational preparation versus liberal education.

Historically, the typical instruction in gerontology appears to have emerged from the liberal education tradition, with faculty members developing an interest in this area and sharing it with their students regardless of the vocational possibilities. As increased knowledge about the process and outcomes of aging developed, gerontology began to take its place as a subfield within such disciplines as sociology, psychology, and biology.

Recently, however, a change has occurred which emphasizes the value of gerontology education in preparing personnel to administer and conduct the service programs which have been initiated through the financial resources of government agencies. This need for increased and improved manpower has led the federal government to provide funding support for the development and conduct of training projects which were designed to relate directly to current planning and programming needs.

The development of age-segregated service programs—those designed to serve primarily or exclusively older people—has encouraged the educational preparation of professionals who are especially knowledgeable and sympathetic to this service delivery system. The needs of the "Aging Network" are often referred to and education of personnel for this system has expanded rapidly. However, in a broader context, the overwhelming size of the aging problem has also had its impact. The financial resources being devoted to the aged, the sheer numbers of persons, and the realization that the future doubtless holds even more of the same have encouraged the continued growth of these instructional programs.

The resulting gerontology education has typically been of an interdisciplinary nature. Although it has developed within a variety of different departments and schools in the institutions of higher education, it generally crosses some disciplinary and professional boundaries. Often, faculty for these instructional endeavors are drawn from several fields. This is not to suggest that there is no focus to these programs. On the contrary, most of them have placed some limitations on their endeavors—such as emphasizing the social science aspects, the biological-medical areas, or the administrative-human service components of the field.

In each case, however, the instructional programs involve a commitment to the area of gerontology beyond the expression of an academic interest. It is this commitment which may separate gerontology from many other areas. Since older people comprise a clear clientele group, a great deal of the reformer's zeal accompanies much of the instruction. This is especially true of new recruits to the field but remains noticeable in the public and private pronouncements of government officials and college faculty.

Gerontology education involves a great deal of variation in terms of the content, faculty, outcomes, curricula, and quality. This should not be surprising in a field that is young and one that is developing from several professional bases. However, it is sometimes difficult to adequately describe the parameters and elements of the field when the diversity seems to overcome the similarities.

One of the most critical areas of diversity is in the view toward whether gerontology should be considered a professional field of its own or whether it is more appropriately conducted as an adjunct to one of the existing professional or disciplinary fields. Some faculty now seem to be attempting to move gerontology instruction toward the autonomy and independence which a profession should have. Others would argue that gerontology is an interest area which can only be adequately developed in connection with one of the existing fields. They maintain that there is no such thing as a practicing gerontologist, but rather only social workers, counselors, administrators, or librarians who have a special interest in the older clientele. Whether the future will see a consistent movement in one way or the other is unclear. But a disagreement about the appropriate status for the area is currently with us.

Because this difference of opinion is so substantial, it seems appropriate to identify the position of the Gerontology Program at the University of Nebraska in this continuing dialogue so that the bias of the writer may be recognized and accurately interpreted. First, at the University of Nebraska, we do not offer a degree in gerontology, nor do we want to develop one at this time. Rather, we prefer to see gerontology as a specialization which a student takes in relation to a professional degree program. However, we do believe that gerontology instruction should be planned in such a way that a sequence of courses meets a series of behavioral objectives identified as being useful to personnel working in the field. Consequently, at Nebraska, the Gerontology Program offers credit courses at the undergraduate and graduate levels which supplement the gerontology offerings of other departments of the University. This provides the capability to "fill the gaps" when other departments' courses do not meet the identified need or are not available because of faculty or resource difficulties. Thus, we function very much like a department having our own faculty and courses, but not offering a degree.

Credentials in Gerontology

One way to view gerontology education is to examine the outcomes of the instructional programs in regard to the credential which is awarded upon completion of a specified amount of course work. Some institutions offer no credential at all for the work that is taken in gerontology. Although the student may receive a degree in another field, there is nothing other than an entry on a transcript which indicates that gerontology has been a part of the program. Oftentimes, the courses which are taken are not ordered into any sequence or combination and are only chosen in regard to a student's interests and professional plans. These institutions are indicating, in effect, that gerontology is not a field of study, but is an interest area which may involve different content for various students.

Other institutions have chosen to offer a prescribed sequence of courses which leads to the award of a credential. This may be a certificate of achievement, a minor within a degree program, a degree major, or a separate degree in gerontology. These credentials would appear to be hierarchical with a certificate requiring less work and knowledge than a minor, a minor requiring less than a major, etc. This may not necessarily reflect reality, however, as some programs offering a minor have only one or two courses which are primarily concerned with gerontology with the remainder dealing with related topics. Thus, there is little comparability of programs and no current manner in which the outcomes can be adequately ascertained.

This means that it is nearly impossible to determine the level of performance which may be expected from a graduate in any of the gerontology programs. A student with a degree in gerontology may have fewer credit hours in the area than does a student with a concentration. Neither is it usually possible to determine the content which has been mastered by students in an Associate Degree Program, a Bachelor's Program, a Master's Program, or a Ph.D. Program. It simply is not possible to know which student has learned what content at what level of mastery.

We currently have no set of performance objectives against which we can compare our students and graduates. This makes it difficult to advise students on their career options. Students are likely to ask, "Is it better to get a degree in gerontology or a degree in another area with a specialization in gerontology?" When we do not know what is included in programs at other schools, it is difficult to offer much useful advice.

This problem is compounded by the lack of clarity in the job field. Since few employers list positions for gerontologists, it is difficult to know what gerontological background is likely to be beneficial in seeking a position. In a small, recent survey that was done at the University of Nebraska, agencies providing services to the aging were not found to be requiring gerontology course work of applicants for positions. They did indicate, however, that if two candidates were approximately equal in experience, preparation, and personal qualities, an applicant who had some gerontology course work would definitely be preferred over one who had no such background.

Outcomes of Gerontology Education

As indicated previously, gerontology education is diverse and consistency among the various programs is difficult to assess. However, those instructional endeavors which are directed toward the preparation of professionals to plan, administer, and serve older people do seem to have some goals which can be assumed to be relevant to most programs.

First, gerontology education is generally expected to develop in the student a commitment to the field of service to older people. Although many persons have an interest and a responsiveness to this clientele group, a long-term professional commitment can only be expected to result from in-depth instruction and study. This prolonged exposure will lead to a substantial integration of content, skill, and attitude and is anticipated to result in a career commitment.

A second outcome of gerontology education is the acquisition of accurate knowledge and understanding of the process of aging and of older people. Much erroneous and biased information about the processes of aging and older people exists in this country; training programs can correct this misinformation and replace it with current and hopefully more positive understanding of the events and developments which affect older people. This knowledge will form the basis on which program planning and implementation decisions are made. If the knowledge and the beliefs which are held about older people are accurate, they may be expected to lead to better programming and to more positive outcomes.

A third result of gerontology education is the extension and modification of professional skills as they relate to the older population. Although each professional field has a set of skills which is taught the student who is preparing for practice, there are many times when these skills need to be modified to be appropriately used in the area of aging. In most cases gerontologists seem to agree that the profession—social work, counseling, law, education—should provide the basic skill instruction, but that the gerontology education should provide the opportunity to modify and adapt those practice skills so that they can be most effectively used to help older people.

A final outcome of gerontology education is the acquisition of a firm grasp of the historical and contemporary legislative and programmatic goals for services to older people. Gerontological activity tends to involve a strong sense of moral indignation about the contemporary situation of older people. The history of developments designed to improve the quality of life of older persons needs to be understood by those who find themselves caught in a whirlpool of daily crises and are unable to gain the needed perspective in order to understand the long-term implication of their work.

Although there are doubtless other outcomes which result from gerontology education, these are especially relevant to the professional relating to the conduct of the current community-based programs for older people. They also seem to clearly carry over to those who are educating these professionals and generating the knowledge on which programs are based.

Structure of Gerontology Education

Gerontology education currently exhibits a wide array of structural arrangements within the various colleges and universities of this country. This diversity has resulted from the differing missions and objectives of the various institutions involved. The first advice which is typically given to faculty members desiring to begin some gerontology education effort is to assess the mission of one's educational institution and determine the activities which relate most clearly to that mission.

Few attempts have been made to analyze the various structures or to propose a series of models which adequately describe the current situation. At the University of Nebraska at Omaha we currently have such a project underway, but we are still several months from completion. In an attempt to share some of our thinking at this preliminary stage, however, it appears that there are at least four factors which must be considered in the description or development of the structure and organization of gerontology education. These are (1) the curricula, (2) the faculty, (3) the administration, and (4) the students of the program. The combination of these four factors can provide some insights to several models of gerontology education structure.

Type I: Intradepartmental Structure. The first structural arrangement for gerontology education is characterized by an intradepartmental organization, one where all course offerings would be concentrated within a single department of the institution. The curriculum in this arrangement typically emphasizes the aspects of gerontology which relate most closely to that host discipline or profession, and the gerontology faculty are usually departmentally based.

Administration of gerontology activities is carried out through the established departmental channels with the chairperson of the host department and the faculty committees having responsibility for curricula, student selection, and faculty assignments. Students enrolled in the program are primarily students of the department and only secondarily students of gerontology. In other words, the gerontology effort is a part of, and completely subject to the authority of the host department; there is little or no autonomy for the program faculty or students provided because they selected gerontology as a special academic area of study.

Type II: Interdepartmental Committee. The second type of arrangement has been developed to facilitate gerontology instruction among several departments. This mechanism provides the basis for cooperation among several departments so that a multidisciplinary educational experience can be offered. The curriculum in this type of structure is composed of a combination of new or modified courses which have been coordinated to provide students a comprehensive view of the field of aging. Faculty working in this structure are primarily members of one or another of the academic departments or professional schools and cooperate with the committee in teaching one or two courses.

Administrative structure of this arrangement is minimal. At most a secretary or administrative assistant facilitates the functioning of the committee and assists in the administrative operation. The admission of students to an interdepartmental committee program generally lies with the committee. It has the power to admit, to advise, and to recommend the awarding of a degree to students who have completed the program. Overall, then, the interdepartmental committee offers a more centralized administrative structure where functions of admission, standards, curriculum, and administration are conducted by the gerontology staff, but faculty appointment, promotion, and tenure remain the prerogatives of the academic departments.

Type III: Center or Institute. The third type of structure also provides for interdepartmental cooperation but introduces a larger and better funded administrative organization to facilitate this interaction. This structure is typically called a center or institute. The curriculum as developed by most centers and institutes is a combination of courses offered by several departments. Although the center typically cannot offer credit courses, it exercises some control over these offerings by developing a concentration or specialization which may culminate in the awarding of a certificate to students completing an appropriate course sequence. The faculty offering gerontology courses for a center or institute are not really responsible to the gerontology center, but rather have their academic home in one of the departments.

The administrative structure of a center is more bureaucratic than collegial. It exists outside all of the university departments with its director often reporting to the academic dean or vice-president. Students may be admitted to two different but complementary programs under this arrangement. Admission to a department is necessary for a degree, but admission to the gerontology center's program may be required for completion of the specialization or certificate. Thus, a dual system of admission and completion of the program is achieved.

Type IV: Department of Gerontology. The fourth type of gerontology structure is a separate department of gerontology which has all of the authority and prerogatives which any other department has. This would include offering of courses, employment of faculty, control of administrative functions, and the selection and instruction of students.

Typically, the curriculum of a gerontology department would include a series of courses which could be selected as a graduation major or minor. In this type of structure, the faculty would have the gerontology department as their primary (or exclusive) academic home. Decisions regarding their rank, promotion, and tenure would be made by the department with other academic units having little or no involvement in the process.

A gerontology department would evidence an administrative structure which is similar to other academic departments. A chairperson would be more common than a director and a variety of faculty committees would indicate collegial governance. Students would be admitted, counseled, instructed, and recommended for graduation by the gerontology faculty. No admission to other academic units would be necessary, and no other unit would be likely to have any specific influence over the credentialing process.

Type V: School of Gerontology. The fifth type of gerontology organization is characterized by the creation of a school of gerontology which recruits and selects its students, has its own faculty, offers majors or degrees, and has its own administrative structure which is equal to the other schools or colleges within the institution. The curriculum would likely be well developed and would provide access to the many facets of the field. Rather than having other departments offer gerontology instruction, the Gerontology School would be likely to select faculty with diverse educational preparation and have this group conduct most or all of the credit instruction. The faculty would have no need for the legitimacy provided by other academic departments, so joint faculty appointments would be less likely to occur unless individuals desired to retain their identification with their "discipline." Decisions on appointment, promotion, and tenure would obviously be the prerogative of the Gerontology School.

Administratively, a school is headed by a dean or director who is assisted by a variety of faculty committees. Within the parameters set by the institution, the School would govern itself. Student recruitment, counseling, instruction, and credentialing would be within the authority of the School.

Implications and Trends

The five structural types of gerontology education do not exhaust the possibilities of organizational arrangements. Some institutions of higher education are likely to combine elements of several of the types while others may be outside all of them. For instance, in some colleges or universities, the instructional thrust relates to the area of field work or of noncredit seminars designed to heighten the student's interest in the field of aging. Some programs have a very tenuous structure which depends primarily upon a few faculty members who have personal interest and commitment to the area.

Perhaps more useful than an assessment of the definitive nature of the suggested structural types are the implications which may be drawn from them for the field. The structure of gerontology education is primarily an indication of the extent of control which the gerontology faculty exerts over the instructional program. The lower numbered types (I) clearly provide the gerontology staff little authority over curricula, faculty, administration, and students. The middle levels (II and III) allow more control over administration and students, but little over curricula or faculty. The upper levels (IV and V) provide control over all aspects of the program. There are those who would assert that only by exercising careful control over the development and operation of gerontology education can the instruction be directed precisely enough so that the graduates of the program will have acquired both the interdisciplinary depth and needed skills for employment in the area of aging. With control vested in several other academic units, the outcome may be neither good sociology, for example, nor good gerontology.

In addition to viewing the types in terms of levels of control, it also appears that the types comprise a series of stages through which gerontology education is moving. The instructional programs which were established ten or more years ago were typically at the less autonomous end of the hierarchy (the lower levels). When first established, they tended to be small programs within large universities and were primarily dependent upon other instructional units. The more recently established endeavors, however, have tended to fall into the middle or upper levels. As the younger, smaller institutions have entered the gerontology area, they have been willing to create new institutes and departments with greater rapidity and ease than has been the case with the larger and more traditional institutions. Thus, control and its accompanying potential for the assurance of consistency and quality may lie primarily with the new programs.

It would not be unique to discover in the future that gerontology has followed the pattern established by other professional fields, beginning within one or two disciplines, growing to encompass aspects of several academic fields, and eventually, establishing a department or school of its own which educates personnel for the profession which has been created. This certainly has been the case with social work, public administration, adult education, counseling, and criminal justice.

Today there are a few indications that gerontology education is moving in this direction, but the trends are inconclusive at best. Most gerontology faculty still consider themselves to be members of their core disciplines; their professional memberships reflect this posture; and they still view gerontology as a subspecialization. However, some of the newer programs, some of the recent graduates, and a few of the more established practitioners are now referring to themselves as gerontologists. The future may well hold more development in this direction.

This may or may not be a desirable outcome. It appears that the result will be to move the field in a vocational/professional direction and away from the more traditional emphasis on gerontology as a portion of liberal education. This seems to be occurring because the federal government is concerned about the training of personnel for its programs and because institutions of higher education have accepted this as the appropriate direction to take. Perhaps it is, but it should result from conscious decisions with a clear awareness of the trade-offs that must result, rather than to accept it by default.

It may be that we are choosing a short-term outcome which will prove to be decisive in the long run. Perhaps the future will include a profession of applied gerontology and a disciplinary area of academic gerontology. I have difficulty seeing the value of that development. A preferred outcome may well be a continued combination of the two areas so that students gain some of the conceptual and personal knowledge as well as the professional skills.

In conclusion, then, gerontology education currently involves a variety of purposes, credentials, and structures within several levels of postsecondary education. It is not currently possible to provide colleges and universities wishing to enter the field with a neat description or plan for the best way to develop a gerontology program. Rather it seems more appropriate for faculty and administrators in these institutions to ask themselves a series of questions regarding their institution's mission, their preferred outcomes, their current resources, and the political realities of their institution. The answers will doubtless differ from one college to the next, but that difference may well prove to be an asset in approaching a field as diverse as gerontology.

References

Donahue, W. Training in social gerontology. In Claude B. Vetter, *Gerontology, a book of readings*. Springfield, Ill.: Charles C. Thomas, 1963.

Hickey, T. The Association for Gerontology in Higher Education—A brief history. Mimeo., 1976.

Orbach, H. *A history of educational development in gerontology*. Paper presented at the Annual Meeting of AGHE, March, 1976.

Major Concerns and Future Directions in Gerontology and Higher Education

Walter M. Beattie, Jr.
Syracuse University

To identify major concerns and future directions in gerontology and higher education presumes that we know where we are and what we are about. The Association for Gerontology in Higher Education's directory identifies 1,275 colleges and universities with curricula and offerings in gerontology. This is an amazing listing which suggests that the battle to establish programs of gerontological education and research within the formal structure of higher education has, to a large degree, been won. However, I would suggest caution. The listing does not assure us of the content, caliber, or quality of such efforts. If we were to assume that 50 percent met some criteria for positive evaluation, this would, indeed, still represent a large number and a major direction in establishing gerontology within higher education.

However, this also begins to raise major concerns. These include the nature and place of content on aging within the particular levels of higher education—two-year, four-year, graduate and postgraduate—as well as within continuing education and adult education programs. It further raises the question as to how much and for whom should such curricula be organized—for vocational as opposed to liberal education. What is the role of higher education in regard to knowledge about and an understanding of aging for the individual and his own growth and maturation throughout the life span, as well as for his role as a citizen and participant in community decision making? What should be the goal and content of education at each level for personal as well as career development, for service as well as for preparation for educators (the trainers of the trainers) and the knowledge builders (researchers of the future)?

We must, therefore, examine major trends in higher education itself and within such an examination, the place of gerontology. Let me identify a few of these trends.

1. We are all aware that the changing age structure of the student body is following the demographic trends for the nation as a whole. In a recent report to the Governor of the State of New York, the Chancellor of the State University of New York noted the increasing age level of students. "Nearly 50 percent of the students in the university are older than the age traditionally associated with collegiate study." This is further borne out by the fact that more than half of all students enrolled in higher education are enrolled on a part-time rather than a full-time basis.

2. The community college movement is going beyond its traditional role as the entry point for some students to higher education, with the provision of general education to task and vocational specific education at the aide and associate degree level. It is further reaching out into a network of community roles and functions beyond those of traditional higher education and in some instances taking on major planning, coordination, and information dissemination roles throughout the communities.

3. The four-year liberal arts education is increasingly mixing its liberalizing goals with vocational goals and in some areas becoming the first professional degree level as, for example, in social work education.

4. Master's professional education is moving toward areas of specialization and concentration with a heavy emphasis on substantive knowledge and skills, rather than those that are more generic.

5. Doctoral education is increasingly providing for more interdisciplinary approaches to research and for scholarly preparation in addition to those which are more disciplinary oriented. Support systems for such education are expanding through interdisciplinary and problem-oriented approaches of the National Science Foundation, the National Endowment for the Humanities, etc.

6. Postdoctoral and postgraduate opportunities are emerging to provide support for persons who have achieved terminal degrees and who are moving toward new areas of scholarly or professional responsibilities.

Within this context the question of gerontology, its organization and its place in higher education, must be viewed. Are career lines to be developed in gerontology per se, that is, as degree programs, as is the emerging trend in some colleges and universities at community college, baccalaureate, and graduate levels? What are the implications of such trends? Is there a core of knowledge exclusive to gerontology or are there cores of knowledge in gerontology related to definable, yet separate, career lines in the field of aging?

Many of us have argued that gerontology requires a multidisciplinary approach and interdisciplinary linkages. Some of us have argued, but not all, that in addition to the multidisciplinary-interdisciplinary framework, there must be disciplinary depth. This latter view stems from a concern that if gerontology is removed from the main streams of research, education, and practice in each of the disciplines, it will become isolated and perhaps suffer from a lack of quality due to its failure to meet the criteria and standards of the root disciplines and professions. This, admittedly involves a philosophical stance as to whether the goal is to build commitments by the more traditional disciplines and professions to aging, or whether a new discipline— gerontology—and a new profession concerned with the application of geron- tological knowledge to the well-being of the elderly is the goal.

The acceptance of one alternative as opposed to the other will have profound implications for the goals and organization of curricula, as well as for the response of higher education itself. I believe this is where we are now with no clear resolution of the difference or, perhaps, no agreement that such a difference, indeed, exists.

Let me now turn to the future. It is my judgment that older persons and knowledge related to gerontology will have a profound effect on the roles and responses of higher education in the immediate decades ahead. The nature of such roles and responses will be dependent, however, on today's decision and responses. These include:

1. There is clear need to establish new administrative structures to deal with adult learners and their advisement, counseling, and service needs. Free or reduced tuition is only a limited response to the educational needs of older adults. This area, unfortunately, has not, in my judgment, been attended to by most universities and colleges. For the most part the older person has to fit into the typical system organized around younger students, who are facing quite different dimensions of concern and decision making than those con- fronting the older student-learner.

2. That faculty must begin to review and revise their views of the learning processes as these are affected by different patterns of intellectual function and organization of information. We must begin to use what we know about the physiological and behavioral changes associated with aging in our own academic houses in regard to the learning environment—physical, psychological, and social—as a way of responding to the new mature student who, indeed, has far different personal resources and characteristics as- sociated with his motivation and goals for learning.

3. For the increasing numbers of younger students seeking careers in work with the aging or preparing themselves for teaching and research careers in gerontology, have we begun to identify career lines and professional- occupation opportunities that currently exist or which are emerging? What kind of advisement, counseling, and guidance system is emerging or should

emerge and what is the character of the knowledge and information which should be available to administrators and faculties in higher education as they respond to students seeking career identification in this emerging field?

4. It is my judgment that, although curricula are expanding, insufficient attention has been given to the continuing education of faculty in the area of their own professional development vis-à-vis aging and in their responsibilities in curriculum development and in the design of courses related to aging. This, I believe, is of critical importance in developing faculty resources with competence and depth in higher education and aging.

5. Finally, the organizational forms for gerontology in higher education—such as institutes, centers, departments, schools, and programs—will, in my judgment, need to be based on the traditions and organizational forms of colleges and universities within particular environments and through past traditions. It will be dangerous to have premature closure as to one approach being more appropriate than another. However, it will begin to force the issue of whether or not gerontology will be a discipline in itself or an area of study, research, and service which is part of other areas of higher education.

In all probability, the future will see a movement toward the development of criteria and standards in the areas of curricula content and organization, faculty, and students. It is my hope that this is not forced prematurely in an area as young as gerontology which has had a history of little more than 30 years. It must not suffer from premature closure and if you will, "hardening of the arteries"; rather, the need is for creativity, the free flow of ideas and their exchange, as well as for a variety of approaches which will provide stimulus to the increasing responses by higher education to gerontology in the immediate decades ahead.

A major concern, important to the future, and essential to consider, beyond the place and organization of gerontology in higher education, is its sources of fiscal support and the manner in which such resources are provided. Time does not permit my discussing fully all aspects or dimensions of this concern. Let me, therefore, merely identify them here and hopefully we can discuss them more fully during later phases of this conference or in future meetings.

1. The need to build gerontology on a hard dollar rather than a soft dollar, grant or contract commitment. Although federal and state resources, as well as private foundation monies have become increasingly available during the past year or two, on a time-limited project or grant basis, sustained support for higher education's responses to aging should be viewed as a legitimate claim on a college's or university's hard dollar budget as are educational and research programs relating to other stages of the life span.

2. The increasing requirement by the Administration on Aging, that career training proposals and other forms of support be reviewed by local Area

and State Agencies on Aging, raises important questions as to the potential constraints and responses of higher education to follow the dollar and move further to task-oriented training.

This is a complex area of concern. I raise it, not because I fail to see a partnership between the academy and society, but rather, because it may lead to unanticipated and undesirable directions in higher education and in government. Creative tensions between higher education and government are essential in my judgment. Dominance of government over higher education and for higher education only to be responsive to government funding will be disastrous. Partnership—yes; dominance—no.

Much of gerontology to date, and the approaches to curriculum development and design, has emphasized knowledge building (research) and education on the basic mechanisms and processes of aging—biological, psychological, and social. For the professions the emphasis has been on the application or translation of such knowledge for practice, social and physical planning, and policy formation. This has been essential and necessary to the development of gerontology in higher education. However, it is not sufficient. It is not enough to know and to do. The critical questions in aging—questions confronting older persons, their families, communities, and society as a whole—is that of meaning or purpose, especially as related to the last third or fourth of the life span.

Each day the question is raised in many forms: What is the purpose of an existence—free of family responsibilities, free of work responsibilities, free of community responsibilities—if time has no structure or meaning? How can we defend payments and reimbursements to persons responsible for nursing homes and long-term care of the aging—if we measure and reimburse only that care which is measured and defined as skilled nursing beds or health related facilities—and not for the other dimensions of care and service that address the less measurable, but perhaps most essential dimensions of the human condition? I, for one, do not believe that science will save us. I, for one, would paraphrase Robert Lynd's "Knowledge for What?" and say "Aging— for What?"

Here, I would suggest, my concern is that we must engage our colleagues from the Humanities, Philosophy, Ethics, Religion, Literature, History—to name a few. These disciplines must begin to reach out to our students (as well as to ourselves) and involve themselves in the central questions involved in aging in the latter fourth of the twentieth century.

Perhaps, if you will permit me to quote from a research prospectus prepared by one of my Syracuse University colleagues, Professor William Melczer, who identifies his fields of competence as Comparative Literature of the late European Middle Ages and the Renaissance, the History of Ideas, and Humanities, you will understand why I identify this area of academic effort in gerontology as a major concern and a much needed future direction.

The rationale for the present research proposal lies in the necessary interaction of the humanities with the social and the physical sciences. Granted the importance of the present day revival of the interest in the aged, the aging process, and old age, these interests have in the main been oriented towards the understanding first, and the betterment later, of the biological, physical, economical, social, and psychological conditions of the aged. Such preoccupations, valid as they are, ought to be complemented by, and balanced with, a concomitant concern for the spiritual and intellectual life of the aged. Standard of life, to have any long-range significance, should go hand in hand with quality of mind. Under quality of mind, though, it is not "culture" or academic education that is meant. Certainly not Kultur with a capital K. Instead, it is the awakening of man's capacity for memory and evocation, the prompting of intellectual pursuits motivated by affective concerns, the fostering of mental activities involving the proto-concerns of positive human behavior—kindness, helpfulness, gregariousness—that constitute the dynamic elements of such a quality of mind. For the mature and the elderly, quality of mind fundamentally buttresses the feeling of togetherness and the feeling of belonging to a single humanity above and beyond historical periods and biological ages.

Our challenge for the future is to design programs in higher education which do not view aging and older persons as merely the objects of study and practice. Our understandings must lead to a clearer view of the meanings and purposes of the latter stages of life in the modern world.

Key Issues Involved in the Growth of Gerontology in Higher Education: A Science in Society Perspective

Fred Cottrell
Miami University

Some of the issues we face grow primarily out of the rapid changes in what people must do to make effective use of science and technology as compared with what the traditional structure of higher education is prepared to teach them.

The day is past when a community of scholars can determine of what higher education shall consist, who will be permitted to provide it and who will receive it. What started as a means to educate people for medicine, law, or the clergy has, with the development of science and technology, proliferated not only to teach the old professions but also prepare for careers in agriculture, mining, engineering, and business as well as education itself. But on a great many campuses preprofessional education as well as advanced graduate work is controlled by the faculty of the Arts College and its attached graduate disciplines in which departmental autonomy is prevalent. This has proved to be so onerous to some innovators that many new branches of knowledge and the creative outgrowths of old disciplines have been cut away and clustered into schools preparing primarily for advanced work in new fields of knowledge. Students there learn to achieve in careers for which the older curricula curricula did not prepare them.

It is now becoming clear to those who select people for jobs that much of what is rewarded by academicians often has little or no relation to successful performance of many things the public demands be done. And many students find that what is being taught is not relevant to achievement in fields in which they wish to work. This has produced a struggle between those who want to impart the "eternal verities" and to advance the traditional wisdom and those who see students abandoning the old sources in favor of means more quickly, surely, and at lower costs, to achieve success in the world outside academia. The demand for this kind of knowledge has become so great that even the most academically prestigious universities have set up graduate schools to teach business, and technical schools such as Cal-Tech and MIT have proved themselves capable of turning out scholars of the highest rank.

Those universities that refuse to accede to the demands of the public that higher education contribute to advances in the solution of problems that trouble them, find it harder and harder to get financial support. Public institutions that depend on the legislatures for funds are rewarded for giving the voter-taxpayer what he seeks, and deprived for their failure to do so. The unwillingness or inability of those who control higher education to find promising solutions to problems, even though that requires them to break through the disciplinary lines that are set up in traditional academia, leads to popular frustration and to the search for effective ways to get done what they want done.

The emergence of new schools prepared to attempt solutions, even at the cost of lower academic prestige, is not primarily a result of a new ideology that demands their creation in order to achieve an ideal system. It develops out of feedback from success in dealing with the problems of people.

The recent development of the academic focus upon older people evidences growing awareness of their special needs and desires, and also shows how higher education is being altered by the effort to use and create new knowledge to that end. Just what part it can play, and will play, will result in part from the nature of the problems old people face. Since higher education is multifunctional, it cannot be expected to ever fit perfectly what is required by the needs and aspirations of older people as they deal with a changing world. But there are a number of different systems, each better or worse than traditional colleges and universities, to solve specific problems. They compete for the opportunity to participate in the action, and have been doing so in increasing numbers.

During most of American history, people assumed that the problems faced by older people were to be solved by the family and local community. During the Great Depression it became obvious that in an urban industrial society this was too great a burden for traditional institutions to successfully cope with. The means once present in the relatively self-subsistent community were inadequate, and the New Dealers set out to use government, which could command the resources of the market and the corporation to redistribute wealth and redirect the flow of goods and services.

The shift in direction of this flow required the appearance of a great new set of servitors, the creation of new jobs for people who had never done them before, the discovery of new techniques not previously taught in the institutions of higher learning, and the ability to anticipate what would be the impact of all these changes on the rest of the American system.

During the Depression Marx and Freud exercised strong influences on the development of change in economics and psychology. The academicians, to the degree that they influenced theory to explain what was going on and what was to be done, used the premises and the arguments their mentors called for. But a great deal of the New Deal was pure unadulterated and unabashed pragmatism. What worked was expanded and what didn't was reversed without apology or explanation. Newer forms of intervention were defended in some institutions of higher education and such innovations as schools of social work flourished.

Politics frequently replaced economics in the determination of remedies. Social workers emphasized children and youth as the strategic points to correct evils. And political economists saw the replacement of old workers by young men as one means to support families of the unemployed. So two new sets of servitors appeared to join medical men as dominant in the bureaucracies that emerged to serve the elders.

Social security and unemployment insurance plus a host of agencies designed to eliminate poverty were expected to deal with low-income people of all ages. Medicine, which has treated all ages in terms of specific diseases, continued to be dominated by the old disciplines that have long been established in the schools of medicine. Those in other agencies dealing with old people noted numerous gaps in medical knowledge and pressed for federal support for research in health sciences.

But when the National Institutes of Health appeared they reinforced not only the existing directions of research, but also the practice of health services delivery. The National Institute of Child Health and Human Development, true to the Freudian influence, concentrated its attention on early development. The changes that occur late in life were, and apparently still are, most often treated as disease entities rather than normal products of long life.

People in various disciplines who came into contact with older people also recognized the interdependence of the factors involved in solving their problems. They set out to build a new set of professions and institutions on a multidisciplinary base. The coterie of interested people that made up the first institutes on aging included specialists in health, housing, psychiatry, social psychology, architecture, anthropology, economics, sociology, political science, recreation, nutrition, social work, and other respectable disciplines and professions. They recognized that older people have needs that involve all these bodies of knowledge in different ways than are required by other sets of age groups. The problem of finding ways to integrate this knowledge is still central to our concern here.

But even in the absence of such a synthesis the problems of elders thrust themselves forward for action. The means to provide income on the basis of need inevitably served the growing number of needy aged. New means of providing medical care to the increasing numbers of old people were created in spite of the active efforts of the powerful AMA to prevent their appearance. Housing for the elderly poor had to be treated differently than that for younger people partly because of the different needs of old and young and in part due to differences in the probability that they would live to pay for it. Older people need different kinds of nutrition, recreation, and transportation than do younger ones. And their growing awareness of these facts has led politicians to attempt solutions even if there were not experts among those delivering higher education to show how these different moves impacted upon one another, and upon the means simultaneously being developed to solve the common problems of both young and old. So the need for synthesis is apparent, even though its solution requires that the impenetrable walls placed around the disciplines by departmental autonomy and the professional monopolies they engender be breached.

The federal government, seeking to make knowledge about aging more effective, frequently found that institutions of higher learning were interested primarily in gaining government support for the perpetuation of the disciplines which had been developed in the past, research to refine and push forward that which they were already equipped to carry on. By and large the universities were discipline-minded while the public was becoming more and more problem-oriented.

Agencies like the Administration on Aging found that money given for research into new fields was being diverted into the support of programs that could hardly be shown to contribute to the immediate solution of the problems of old people, particularly as those problems were exacerbated by the results of other government policies. The Congress increasingly heard demands that what was done for old people at government expense be demonstrated as helping old people, not others who were ripping them off. So government has been seeking new avenues to learn what has worked and what has not.

Often that knowledge came, not from institutions of higher learning, but from practitioners in contact with the elderly, from administrators responding to directives from Washington, in terms of their effects on old people and programs supposed to help them. Studies of those engaged in those programs found that the universities were in many cases continuing to follow old curricula that had become less and less useful. For example, social workers were less and less able to do case work, more and more they were involved in administration, in public law, in accounting, and so on, yet many entered the field because of its promise that they would work directly with deprived people and spent most of their time learning things that would permit them to do so effectively in spite of declining opportunities. Yet autonomy and tenure perpetuated the system.

At the outset of the development of gerontology as a synthetic field there were few who had the knowledge to teach what the emerging occupations demanded. Some institutions saw that need and set out to provide the rudiments as they discovered them to people poorly equipped to carry on at higher levels. These efforts are now paying off as a body of secondary knowledge is developed and passed on to those in the field.

The emergence of the whole junior and community college movement has modified the need for advanced faculty to be engaged primarily in teaching. Those in more advanced higher education can increasingly teach what they have learned through research to the faculty and to administrators of the new branches, who in turn will be able to supply trained personnel for the expanding needs of the elderly, and do it at a lower cost, right in the communities where people are likely to be employed.

This move to respond in terms of regional differences, apparent in the creation of the AAAs [Area Agencies on Aging], means that those engaged in teaching and research must become highly eclectic in the methods and materials they use. Abstract principles do not solve cases. So a move in the direction of establishing fixed standards and techniques as a qualification for professional advance needs to be given extensive scrutiny. We have no monopoly on learning or teaching about aging. Universities will have to deal with the facts of life or lose control over research and teaching that is not best served by the traditional academic system. Multidisciplinary knowledge has been given a low rating in academia. Promotions and opportunity for further research go to those who advance further into the narrow defiles of the disciplines. But the people who supply the wherewithal to solve the complex situations they face are impatient. They have been turning in great numbers to contract research, research carried out by problem-solving foundations, even to unions and other organizations with their own axes to grind. Any effort just now to put a limit on those whom we are ready to call Gerontologists is abortive. We need the help of everybody who has anything to contribute to the solution of problems of the elderly.

Major Concerns and Future Directions in Gerontology and Higher Education: A Perspective from Our Knowledge Base

Martha Storandt
Washington University

I have noted a wave of anti-intellectualism in gerontology. I observe a flavor of emotionally laden humanism and altruism in our daily activities, as well as in the workings of policy-determining bodies, program committees, and other components of many of our gerontological organizations. Although I value the ethic of social justice for all members of our society, the aged in particular, I also value the search for and development of knowledge. Without a solid knowledge base, humanism can be just as tyrannical as authoritarianism. We who are members of institutions of higher education should be especially sensitive to this and, perhaps, better aware than many others of its potentially disastrous effects.

Let me give you an example. Many gerontologists favor the elimination of mandatory retirement policies. We are well aware of the human suffering that such policies produce and the waste that can arise when productive, wise, capable individuals are eliminated from our work force on the basis of their chronological age alone. However, how many of us have given serious thought to the consequences of the elimination of mandatory retirement? How many of us have thought about the impact on younger workers? How many of us have thought about the stagnation that might arise in the factories and businesses of our country, not to mention the universities and colleges, if one individual held the same position of employment for 50 or 60 years? What about the impact of such stagnation upon that individual? What would it be like to do the same thing for 60 years? Or even 20 years? How many of us have thought of the "workaholics" who would never have an opportunity to put their lives in order and prepare for death because they would be able to deny its inevitability until the final moment by continuing to shut out all else in life but their employment? How many of us have thought that large segments of our society may in fact enjoy retirement, even if we professionals see it in a negative light? How many of us have thought of the discontinuities which would arise if positions were filled hurriedly and without prior planning after the death of one individual, rather than in a planned manner in preparation for the retirement of that individual?

Thus, I would recommend that before we endorse and work for a policy that appeals to us on an emotional level we take a much closer look at all the parameters involved. We need an environmental impact statement based on data, not a rallying to the cause, based on beliefs, armchair theories, and our own emotional needs.

Let me give you another example from my own discipline. Many of us have long decried the lack of interest in the old on the part of the clinical psychologist. I used to berate my colleagues who worked with children and young adults for their lack of knowledge about, and interest in, the old. And, there's no denying that lack of interest, based on several recent surveys and other data gathering devices.

However, before clinicians can treat the emotional problems of the aged, they must know what treatment to apply. It may well be that techniques of psychotherapy appropriate to the young are inappropriate or ineffectual with respect to the aged. Further, some of the more common psychiatric problems faced by the old are related to organic changes in the brain. Psychiatry and clinical psychology are largely impotent in the treatment of such disorders, having focused in the past upon the treatment of "functional" rather than organic syndromes. What good is it to have a practitioner who has nothing to practice? Before we can develop extensive training programs for clinical psychologists, psychiatrists, or other mental health workers in gerontology, we must first spend our resources upon developing a knowledge base that these people can use. Thus, the first order of business is to train and nurture research clinicians, not practitioners in the same old model.

Now this is the point at which many of you may be ready to turn off your hearing aids, go to sleep, or otherwise leave the field. So many gerontologists want to do good works but are uninterested in finding out what those good works are. I am appalled by the poor quality of the research I hear reported at many of our national meetings and see published in some journals. I am even more appalled by the quality of the papers that are submitted for presentation and publication. How can we train people to provide services to older adults if we do not really know what services are worthwhile and what services are just someone's pipe dream? In order to do this, these services must be evaluated, theories must be put to the test of experimental, scientific verification or rejection. Evaluation does not mean that some authority thinks the program is good. It means that the effectiveness of the program has been demonstrated in a public, repeatable, objective manner. The experimental group must be compared to the control group, if you will. Or, subjects must be tested both before and after they have received the recommended services or treatments to see if any real benefits have arisen. Further, evaluation must be objective. Ratings must be made either by individuals uninvolved in the treatment itself, or in a "double blind" paradigm where the evaluator does not know what treatment was received by the client or patient.

It takes many years to learn research methodology and statistics as they apply to gerontology. I do not expect every person interested in aging to become a statistician. However, I do expect each and every program on aging in an institution of higher education to have some expertise in gerontological research methodology. Someone whose primary responsibility is to serve as a resource both to the university or college and to the community as a whole to make sure that all our new and wonderful programs for the aged are really wonderful—not just new.

However, I do not want to let the rest of you off the hook so easily. I expect your methodology expert to do everything in his or her power to educate all of you in the scientific method as it applies to gerontology. I charge you all to become critical consumers of research. Do not buy the product unless it measures up. Know the criteria of good research and apply those criteria, no matter how much you would like to ignore them on an emotional basis.

Further, I expect funding agencies to do their part in educating us all with respect to quality research in gerontology. Research funds should be awarded only on the basis of scientific merit. Quality peer review of proposed research is an absolute necessity. And by quality peer review, I mean that those who serve to screen and evaluate proposed research must be knowledgeable in both the content and methodology of the area. Detailed evaluations should be returned to the researcher, outlining the ways in which the proposed research could be improved. I realize this places a great burden upon review panels, but they must take their jobs seriously. It is not just an honor—it is a responsibility. I also charge them to try to submerge their own values and priorities with respect to research content. This is a very difficult task; I can only ask that they try.

Finally, the various national and local professional organizations related to the study of aging can take an active role in providing research education to their membership. Instead of another symposium or paper session on institutionalization versus home care, on locus of control, on chronic brain syndrome, or even on cognitive changes with age, we should have sessions over the next few years on the appropriate methodology for investigating these areas.

I have seen more enthusiasm and sparks generated in the past two or three years at those meetings where cross-sequential methodology was the subject of discussion than at any other meetings I have attended. Whatever the final outcome of those discussions, they are serving a useful function in bringing methodological issues to the attention of the gerontological community.

This remedial methodological education—through our journals as well—should be a short-term project. We should not have to focus on it forever, in an educational sense. If we are at all effective in transmitting knowledge, one to another, gerontologists will become more sophisticated in research techniques as the years go by and will train their students at the undergraduate and graduate level so we will not have to do a patch-up job later.

During its brief history AGHE has represented, to a very large extent, those educational programs in gerontology which are predominantly concerned with training individuals in disciplines and career fields related to social gerontology. We have relatively little representation from educational programs in the biomedical professions, the physical sciences, or the humanities as they relate to the aged. This is most likely due to the fact that the number of gerontological programs in these fields is very small. I do not see it as a policy of exclusion on the association's part.

Within the past year AGHE has made a concerted effort to try to broaden its representation and to search out and invite representation from, for example, medical education programs. We have been mildly successful, in terms of the symposium presented at the Gerontological Society's 1976 Annual Meeting, and in terms of the participation at our present meeting here in Tucson of a number of representatives from the Veterans Administration's Office of Academic Affairs, Regional Medical Educational Centers, and Geriatric Research, Education, and Clinical Centers. However, I see as one of our future goals continued efforts to "gerontologize" programs of higher education in these underrepresented fields. For AGHE to truly represent Gerontology in Higher Education, we must recognize all of higher education. We cannot limit our association's activities to issues which intimately and directly concern our present and traditional membership. We must take a broader view, in terms of an organized effort to represent all aspects of higher education which may have some impact on the condition of the older adult.

Certainly one aspect of such a broader view would be a concerted effort on the part of our membership committee to seek out new member institutions with programs in gerontology in these underrepresented disciplines and professions. However, AGHE must also assist each representative from present member institutions to expand those institutions' involvement in gerontology. Many of us come from universities with many diverse departments and schools. Are we truly representing all segments of our universities, or just our own program or department?

Each of AGHE's committees can place high on its list of priorities some activity which will assist us in this expansion process. For example, the executive committee may find it appropriate to recommend that AGHE form some sort of liaison with national organizations of underrepresented professions—nursing, medicine, biochemistry, human engineering. Our public policy committee, as overworked as it already is, may expand its concerns to include policy issues as they relate to the training of, for example, physicians, nurses, nurses' aides, and other health care delivery personnel. Our program committee may wish to continue setting aside a portion of the annual meeting to deal with educational issues in these underrepresented disciplines. The Association could also consider applying for program time at national meetings of organizations which deal with educational issues in these fields.

To summarize, one long-range future goal of AGHE may be the nurturance of gerontological education programs in all disciplines and professions which impinge upon the older adult, with a targeting of educational programs in the health care field as a high priority item within this long-range goal.

Let me now shift to the issue of the quality of the education in gerontology. I am in real conflict on this issue. In some ways I favor anarchy, or an absence of laws and supreme power. How sweet life would be if we could all do our own thing! Of course, this naive dream requires that all others go about doing their own thing and not interfering with us. It also requires that we all do our own thing to the best of our ability.

Thus, philosophically, I am not generally in favor of a set of formalized rules relating to the quality of gerontological education, nor am I in favor of an elaborate accreditation procedure. This is the anarchist in me. It also represents the pragmatist. I recognize that rules and regulations, accreditation committees and boards lead to a staggering bureaucracy, stifling red tape, and much money spent on something which in all likelihood may be ineffectual in accomplishing its goals. Formalized rules, such as state regulations dealing with nursing homes, all too often have to deal with entities such as the number of fire escapes, width of the doors, and the number of nurses on duty at any one time, rather than the quality of those fire escapes, what goes on in the rooms those doors lead to, and the effectiveness of those nurses when they are on duty.

I also recognize that the gerontological educational programs we wish to see become quality programs must operate within the fiscal constraints faced by all educational programs. If a given gerontology program must be allotted a specific amount of additional money in order to bring it up to those standards required by some accrediting procedure, other programs within that institution might be given priority and the gerontology program phased out.

So what's the solution to this problem of our desire to provide quality education in aging, on the one hand, but the realities of accrediting procedures on the other hand? First, I recommend that at this time we do not set up any formal guidelines, rules, or regulations dealing with accreditation, program quality, or the like. However, I do strongly recommend that within our organization we place high on our list of priorities the development of methods for making sure that the educational programs in gerontology represented in our organization are of the highest quality. If they are not that way now, we must set about developing the mechanisms for helping them to become that way. In other words, I want to socialize rather than legislate quality into our gerontology programs.

I call for the designation of an AGHE Task Force to be charged with developing the mechanisms to accomplish this goal of quality gerontological education. These mechanisms must leave sufficient latitude for the development of diverse programs, examining aging from many points of view. The one thing we don't want to do is force everyone into the same mold. Such a task force would have a long and difficult job, but I am afraid that if we do not do it for ourselves, we will be faced with an imposed structure of regulations from without—a set of rules and procedures which will, in the end, stifle the creativity and diversity sorely needed in gerontology.

What shall be done about the many new people who are coming to gerontology? I say welcome them with outstretched arms, train them to be good gerontologists and put them to work. The big problem will be to train them—there is plenty of work. I suggest that one of the challenges facing AGHE in the near future is the nurturance of training programs for professionals who, in midcareer, or any other part of their career, wish to take on the added specialty of aging. I do not think the presently available methods of dealing with this issue are adequate or effective. These methods tend to involve the continuing education credit, brief workshops of questionable quality and long-term gains, and postdoctoral training programs in research. All of these have their problems.

The current mechanism of postdoctoral fellowships is for researchers only and does not touch on the issue of training the educator, the service provider, the clinician. We need a fresh, new look at alternative mechanisms—beyond that of continuing education credits—for retraining professionals newly involved in gerontology and for updating the knowledge base of gerontologists long involved in their particular discipline or field. The academic sabbatical might serve as a model in some instances. However, given that the potential gerontologist can find some method of convincing his or her employer to provide the leave, are we prepared to give these individuals the kind of training they want and deserve?

And if we are going to have short-term training, whatever happened to the concept of evaluation? Before someone is given credit for being able to do something, in most cases we ask them to demonstrate that they can indeed perform the task. Before a driver is allowed to venture out on the highways and streets of our country, that driver must take a written as well as a performance test, so that he or she can be certified as a qualified driver. Before a certified accountant can do a company's books or prepare your tax return, he or she must pass a written examination. What's wrong with requiring those who attend our brief training seminars, workshops, or institutes to pass some sort of examination so that they, and we, may determine if they have absorbed, in some fashion or another, the information presented to them? These individuals would then at least be aware of their own shortcomings and knowledge gaps. And we would know where we are doing a good job and where we are falling down.

I am sure there are at least two practical problems with such a program of evaluation. One, as the purveyors of such educational experiences, we may be put to shame when some of our students flunk the final exam. Also, the students may refuse to come to our educational activities and the short-term training business may not flourish. All of the resistance to evaluation, however, will be carefully camouflaged as a philosophical opposition to treating people as if they are not mature enough to take responsibility for their own learning.

I have been talking about the education and training of individuals of all ages who intend to make a career of the study of aging. Now I would like to speak to the issue of the older adult—the subject of all our interests—in the institution of higher education. I see many of the programs, policies, and treatment techniques we currently prescribe for older adults as backwards. We are faced with people in distress and we try to devise some means of meeting their needs, after those needs have become acute. Why don't we try some prevention?

It seems to me that the original example I gave today about mandatory retirement would become a moot issue if the members of our society were to value leisure. No one would be concerned about mandatory retirement policies, if people did not fear the loss of their jobs but instead looked forward to retirement with expectation and desire. Why haven't we been involved in educating people to use the last years of their lives in a meaningful manner? Of all the failings of gerontology, this is perhaps the most serious. We have focused on training people for careers as service providers to the elderly, rather than on training the population as a whole to deal meaningfully and successfully with old age so that the need for service providers is reduced.

There have been some scattered efforts to provide educational programs for older adults in our colleges and universities. These have not been extensive and little effort has been made to evaluate their benefits. Thus, I would return to my original theme requesting an emphasis upon evaluation of our efforts—this time with respect to educational programs for, not about, older adults.

At the same time we must ask whether all educational efforts directed towards older adults belong in institutions of higher education? Might not some of them be better carried out by other institutions in our society? For example, why haven't we involved the mass media to a greater extent in educating the population as a whole, and older adults in particular, about aging? I have recently seen two public service spot announcements which dealt with the meaning of life in the postretirement years. Both were accurate, from a gerontologist's point of view, but I have no idea of how wide an audience they reached or how effective they were with respect to the general population. Those universities with educational programs in mass media communications should be drawn into our gerontological community and we should put them to work in terms of preventive education for the later years of life. For example, what are the most effective means of reaching large segments of the older television viewing audience? Should we use documentaries, soap operas, or a Lawrence Welk format?

As was suggested several years ago at one of the regional planning meetings for the last White House Conference on Aging, perhaps what we need is an Elder's Television Workshop which will do for the education of mature and older adults the same thing that Sesame Street and The Electric Company have done for early childhood education. Therefore, although I have asked this group today many questions, and have not supplied many answers, I would like to ask just one more before I close. This one may be the most fun to answer and will probably carry with it the biggest payoff. "Can you tell me how to get to Sesame Street?"

Education in a Human Services Context:
A View from the Research Literature

Tom Hickey
University of Michigan

Research on human services and delivery systems for aging in the area of education reflects two issues: (1) education for enhancing the quality of life through the improved delivery of human services to the aged; and, (2) education throughout life as a human service of our society for positive adult development. From an educational perspective, the first of these is based on a long tradition of entry-level and continuing professional and technical education for practitioners. The latter focuses on the ideal of continuing human development through the process of lifelong learning. From a research perspective, however, these two are closely linked to the state-of-our-knowledge about the processes of aging and about changing age cohorts of adults. In effect, both deal with the education of adults: on the one hand, training adults to provide optimal care and services for the aging; and on the other hand, education in many subject areas to facilitate optimal growth and development throughout life. Thus, educational research in this context implies a dual focus on knowledge gaps in understanding all dimensions of the learning process, and on the continuing application of what we know about adults and adult learning to the education of adults—whether it be for lifelong learning or for the improvement of services to other adults.

The purpose of this paper then is twofold: to summarize the state-of-the-art in those areas which seem to have the greatest relevance to research on human services and delivery systems in education; and to note the gaps and recommend research priorities which emerge from this discussion. A major focus of this paper will be on research areas which will reflect gaps in our knowledge generation and utilization. The three areas which provide the greatest contribution to this state-of-the-research are adult learning, adult/lifelong education, and human services education and training.

The Application of Adult Learning Research

Any attempt to design and implement educational programs in gerontology must take into account what is known about adults as learners. It has long been assumed that intellectual abilities decline with age and that older adults were incapable of learning. This notion has been challenged from an applied perspective by professionals working with community groups of old people, and from a research perspective with the formulation of life-span developmental research strategies using designs other than the traditional cross-sectional method (Baltes, 1968; Schaie, 1965). The realization that the cross-sectional method confounds age-related changes with historical changes in intellectual performance has led many researchers currently to reconsider the learning capacity of adults. And, in fact, recent research has not found this steady decline, perhaps suggesting that decline may be more indicative of cultural-historical change than true ontogenetic change. It appears that when we compare the old (who have not had the educational advantages of younger cohorts) to the young, the young perform better. Thus, the aged may be obsolete in their performance rather than impaired or in a state of decline. It remains important both to apply what is known about current adult cohorts and to plan for the possibility of adjustments with subsequent cohorts, as we plan and design adult educational programs—either in a lifelong learning or a human services context.

Another significant contribution which has led to a reconsideration of adult learning capacities has been the application of Cattell's (1963) conceptualization of the fluid and crystalized dimensions of intelligence to research with adults. As Baltes and Labouvie (1973) pointed out, the traditional intelligence tests are nondevelopmental in nature and fail to differentiate between dimensions that may increase or decrease with age. Research by Horn and Cattell (1966, 1967) has indicated that one type of intelligence called fluid intelligence exhibits a steady decline from adolescence onward, whereas another type, crystallized intelligence, shows an increase well into old age. The finding that adults are superior in the experiential domain may have tremendous implications for intergenerational learning situations. Furthermore, there may also be potential for modifying the decrement of the fluid component (Plemons, Willis, and Baltes, 1975).

Although it is now evident that older adults are more capable of learning than our negative stereotypes led us to believe previously, it is important to realize that big differences between generations or cohorts do exist in terms of their abilities. All learning research makes the assumption that the underlying learning process is reflected on overt performance; that is, it is assumed that performance on learning tasks is an adequate measure of competence. Therefore, it is necessary to consider factors which may influence performance.

Woodruff and Walsh (1975) discussed and summarized the impact of noncognitive factors such as task meaningfulness, overarousal, and rate of stimulus pacing on adult learning performance. Research has shown that adults have very little interest in the typical nonsense syllable or paired associate task (Botwinick and Storandt, 1974; Hultsch, 1975), and that when given more relevant versions of these tasks, their performance improves (Hulicka, 1967). This motivational component of learning should be an important consideration for educators; and it points to the necessity for meaningful subject matter to insure optimal learning. These data also suggest that we may underestimate old people's competence on the basis of performance measures.

A series of studies by Eisdorfer and his colleagues concluded that adults were more aroused than younger persons as indicated by the level of free fatty acid in the blood, and by the effects of an arousal-blocking drug on performance on a serial learning task (Eisdorfer, Nowlin, and Wilkie, 1970; Powell, Eisdorfer, and Bogdonoff, 1964). At a very basic level, these findings attest to the problems that stressful or anxiety-producing situations may cause for adults in the learning context. One related consideration is the ecological environment in which learning is to occur. It is necessary to determine which settings are least stressful and best approximate ideal learning conditions. It is also necessary to look more systematically at other noncognitive areas (e.g., personality, motivation) within this framework.

Canestrari (1963) and Monge and Hultsch (1971) have shown that older people who were given more time to process and to respond to paired associate tasks utilized the extra response time and subsequently improved their performance. The adaptability of self-paced or programmed learning to adult education would be one way of reducing performance deficits due to speed. Further potential lies in the use of operant techniques and practices which have been successfully used in increasing the performance speed of adults (Hoyer, Labouvie, and Baltes, 1973).

Even if these noncognitive factors are controlled, the adult still does not perform as well as younger subjects. This suggests that there are cognitive variables which also influence their performance (Woodruff and Walsh, 1975). Eisdorfer (1965) found that, given a longer time to study materials, adults performed better, suggesting a cognitive processing deficit. Also, using mediational techniques for remembering word pairs has enabled adults to increase their retention (Canestrari, 1968). Hultsch (1969) found that adults use organizational strategies in memory tasks less efficiently than younger subjects, although when they are instructed in how to organize material, they are capable of doing so and their performance improves. Another important finding of this study was the differential results for high and low verbal adults, the former performing almost as well as younger subjects. This is indicative of the nature and wider range of individual differences in adulthood compared to those in childhood. These need to be carefully considered in planning for many adults in a single educational setting or program.

Woodruff and Birren (1972) reported that older individuals performed as well if not better than younger subjects on a biofeedback task. On the basis of these data (and a more recent study by the senior author) it has been suggested that adults may have superior internal awareness; and Woodruff and Walsh (1975) discussed the implications this may have at a time when self-awareness is highly desirable. It is worthwhile to consider possible applications of brain wave control to information processing and other dimensions of learning. Other implications may lie in the application of this knowledge to the area of affective education as advocated by Looft (1973). Continued exploration of adults' superior capabilities may be useful in the attempt to diminish the negative attitudes of others toward adults as learners as well as those of the elderly themselves toward education.

In summary, recent and currently emerging cognitive and noncognitive areas of adult learning research provide a basis for applied research and demonstration programs in adult education. The future research direction appears to be towards externally valid learning materials (for adults) in a relevant or meaningful context. The materials and the context could reflect either a human services or avocational/lifelong learning goal. The demonstrations themselves should be specific in measuring such variables as cultural-historical change, crystallized intelligence, mediational factors in performance, and the physiological components which relate both to motivation and to performance.

Adult and Lifelong Education Research

The growth and development of the adult and lifelong education movement in this country during recent years has been phenomenal. The Carnegie Commission on Higher Education strongly encouraged colleges in this direction, suggesting a much broader intergenerational focus in curriculum and student body (Scully, 1973). Entire university and college systems have recently redefined their educational missions in terms of a commitment to lifelong learning (Hesburgh, Miller, and Wharton, 1973). In fact, new agencies and funding structures have emerged to launch programmatic demonstrations of adult education and lifelong learning programs (e.g., Fund for the Improvement of Postsecondary Education). An official recognition of this movement occurred with the annual meeting of the National University Extension Association in 1975, which had as its theme, "The New Majority in Higher Education." This theme was based on a national statistic reflecting that slightly over 50 percent of the student body in higher education today are beyond the traditional college student age of 18–25 years.

Therefore, there seems to be little question about the growth and development of adult and lifelong educational programs as an emerging priority human service of our society. In many ways the educational domain provides one of the most optimistic outlooks for aging and gerontology in this country. As noted at the 1971 White House Conference on Aging, ". . . education itself is essentially an affirmative enterprise. . . . [It is] based on the assumption that it will lead to something better in the lives of those participating . . . that older persons are capable of a constructive response to educational stimulation" (WHCOA Report, Vol. II, 1971). In effect, the educational movement has proceeded on a positive basis, whereas adult learning research has been somewhat cautiously attempting to disprove cognitive decline and various age-related incapacities.

While the education movement is itself essentially an affirmative one, nevertheless, there should be much concern about the lagging state-of-the-research which encompasses this movement—research which both leads to program design and emerges from program outcomes. The main characteristic of adult education research seems to be that there is so little of it. An exhaustive review of the literature and research articles in this field reveals three general types of information: (1) "think-type" pieces reflecting policy and program development issues as well as broad overviews of adult, lifelong, and continuing education needs and accomplishments; (2) reports of successful—although typically idiosyncratic—case histories and individual programs; and (3) demographic-type survey research reports of people, programs, needs, accomplishments, etc. The last of these provides a somewhat useful data base for program planning; and the first two types of articles seem to generate new ideas, as well as to reinforce the forward progression of adult education. However, substantive theoretical frameworks and good empirical data (other than head counts and percentages) are generally absent from this literature.

The research chapter in the latest *Handbook of Adult Education* (Smith, Aker, and Kidd, 1970) begins with the somewhat sobering statement: "Two of the more perplexing words in the jargon of the adult educator are the terms program and evaluation." The same chapter concludes quite candidly that research is largely neglected in adult education for two reasons: Programs lack measurable objectives and outcomes; and decision makers ascribe little priority to research and program evaluation (Boyle and Jahns, 1970). This presents a somewhat appalling picture when one considers that it is the clear responsibility in higher education today for all academically based programs to devise a strong theoretical base which carries methodological implications for program evaluation.

Moreover, an additional dimension of the gap here, as noted at the 1971 White House Conference on Aging (WHCOA Report, Vol. II, 1971) and many times since then, is that there is no single unit in the federal government responsible for systematic or programmatic education for aging (which should include educational research).

An obvious task here is to bridge the research gap between the laboratory of adult learning and the real demographic context of lifelong education with a theoretical and empirical base. For example, there are many educational implications to be derived from a life-span development perspective— especially from examination and program application of cohort differences. There is an experientially based predisposition for education and lifelong learning which seems to increase with each succeeding age cohort of adults; yet this is not typically reflected in program design. The medium of television as an educational intervention has apparently kept pace with the technical and hardware research; yet the somewhat obvious cultural-historical differences in socialization from television have received little consideration in educational programming. The "Future Shock" syndrome of rapid obsolescence combined with increasing amounts of leisure time has been reflected in the quality and availability of continuing, avocational, and activity-type courses and programs; yet the cohort differences in values and in attitudes toward work, leisure, family, and life style are only minimally considered.

Some people say that the principle fault of adult education—both its programs and research—is in its categorization and treatment of adults as children. This is not necessarily a useful generalization. It might be closer to the point to say that adulthood cannot be characterized or defined unidimensionally; and thus, education for different stages and purposes throughout adulthood must necessarily differ. Lifelong education is a process, and not a stage like secondary or higher education. One of the more distinguished leaders in this field has stated that, "Adult education will emerge as a full-fledged field only when its master practitioners achieve the ability to apply alternative processes, choosing in each case the one which best meets the requirements of the situation" (Houle, 1973). Education for aging then must be based on research which will generate empirically based, discrete choices and alternatives which can be systematically applied, measured, and replicated.

Research in Education and Training
for Human Services

The past 10 years have seen an impressive growth in the number of professionals trained for applied careers in aging. This growth can be attributed to a number of things, although principally to two continuing events: the emerging "critical mass" of gerontologists in major universities and centers of education; and the annual appropriations for the implementation of the Older Americans Act, which have included limited support for education and training. The former event is itself a part of the latter, as well as a growth function of various NIH-supported education and training programs for gerontology. The impressive growth of this field, however, leaves no room for complacency, as manpower needs have been projected to double during the period of 1973–1978 alone (Chiles, 1973). As many have pointed out, the need for training still far surpasses our accomplishments in this area. The continuing decline in available funds for training is a serious concern.

A comparatively recent development in this area is the allocation of Title IV funds directly to the states for short-term and in-service training, in addition to university-based career training and education programs. Decisions about the use of the available funds for short-term training have resulted in many differences of opinion about priorities and the value of these programs. There is concern, for example, that some training is limited in scope to deal only with existing service program mandates (e.g., Titles III and VII). As service needs change, will these providers have the more generic competency to deal with new issues and needs? Similarly, many short-term training programs do not seem to take into consideration changing age cohorts. As Neugarten and others have pointed out, our currently held conceptions of the elderly very frequently represent that segment of the population which is now over 70 years of age.

The implications of this movement for a research strategy in education as it relates to human services delivery are important. For example, in a tight economy—and one with few available resources for education for gerontological human services delivery—we are beginning to ask some key research questions: What kind of professionals have been trained? Who should now be trained? What kind of educational and training programs have the greatest priority? What is the best educational process? Can we specify the impact of our educational programming on human services delivery? Are those trained now working in aging-related positions? To date, most research in human services training has been of the *product evaluation* type (i.e., how many people were trained to conduct what specific service in which setting or program function). Research in education for human services should begin with answering the questions previously raised. *Process evaluation*, using quasi-experimental models and time-series observations, should be directed towards what happens in the relevant context of learning for human services delivery to older adults. In effect, the degree-of-fit between the *substance of career training* (both in-service and preparatory) and *effective career activities* must be examined systematically.

In two recently published papers, suggestions have been made for delineating program content into three types: *information transmission*, *skill acquisition*, and *attitudinal change* (Connelly, 1975; Hickey, 1975a). Content differentiations such as these provide an easier framework both for assessing program outcomes and for examining the degree of congruence between staff performance and service delivery objectives. The previously mentioned learning research and a number of studies from the educational psychology domain provide means for effectively transmitting information. The intervention and group process literature suggests ways for teaching skills; and emerging studies delineating the attitudes of practitioners should begin to suggest some measurable educational objectives. In another paper, Zerbe and Hickey

(1975) have also recommended that some training programs can be better evaluated in terms of change measures with the client population—in this case the effectiveness of a Self-Maintenance Skills training program was determined from a maintenance-status index of patient behaviors.

In addition to underlining the importance of applied learning research for human services, gerontologists have repeatedly emphasized that no funding mechanism exists for such research. The educational interventions reported by Connelly, Hickey, and others have been based on short-term projects funded to train large numbers of service providers. For the most part, neither the funding sources nor the service agencies have been interested in the research design, the learning process, or the educational context.

In order to bridge the gap between the learning laboratory and the human services learning context, there must be a collaborative process. The goals and objectives of the service program must be incorporated within both the program design and the research hypotheses. On the one hand, practitioners have been asking for training which is both relevant and quickly delivered. On the other hand, researchers and educators are saying that relevance and effectiveness cannot be determined objectively by means of rapidly delivered, idiosyncratic, or charismatic programs. It is again the training-education dichotomy which Weg has repeatedly mentioned; and it is the same problem which afflicts adult education in general—i.e., minimal research is generated due to the absence of an appropriate theoretical framework and because good program outcomes are not carefully determined in advance. On the one hand, ad hoc training for human services demands our support. At the same time, however, a human services strategy demands that relevant research utilization for delivery systems be collaboratively combined with known theoretical and empirically based frameworks for education.

Research Deficiencies and Recommendations

The brief description of research priorities and recommendations which follows is largely defined by the state-of-the-field and by the definitions of the National Institute on Aging—as delineated in the "Research on Aging Act of 1974" (Public Law 93-296). Broadly stated, the primary research intent of the Institute is to promote aging research and to conduct scientific studies to measure the interaction of aging and human services programs and activities. Therefore, our priorities in this paper are the applications of the known learning process variables to adult learning contexts and programs, and the implications of aging and changing age cohorts for education research and for the education of human service providers. Moreover, the emphasis here is on bridging basic and applied components which—when previously considered for funding—have been viewed as separate entities. In addition, the serious gap in research methodologies and methods of learning assessment in naturalistic settings must be dealt with at the outset as a high priority. In brief, education research on human services and delivery systems for aging must focus on *meaningful content for adults in a relevant context and the methodology for assessing that interaction.*

The literature suggests five areas in which immediate research is needed. Each of these areas should represent a sustained programmatic thrust of at least five years duration which would include both narrowly defined, one-dimensional demonstration projects and multi-stage/year studies— especially in the areas of methodological definition and development. Priority should be given to projects which combine demonstrated research expertise in learning application and research utilization for human services, with relevant contexts.

1. The Application of Noncognitive Research Findings to Naturalistic Settings. Given the extensive exploration in the laboratory, it is now necessary to apply these findings and to research these same phenomena in actual learning situations. For example, specific areas of psychobiology and psychophysiology have suggested both deficits and strengths of adults. We must consider ways to apply findings in the areas of pacing, biofeedback, and arousal. We need to create supportive and meaningful learning environments to improve motivation and to test the effectiveness of the application of such findings. Other research considerations could include having the elderly participate in the design of their own programs, to assure personal relevance and perhaps to reduce unnecessary stress. This can be further enhanced by the utilization of self-paced and programmed learning curricula as alternative means of instruction. Previous adult education research has inferred various motivational factors from types and numbers of programs and courses attended. Research now should be directed towards the sustaining affective components of participation in an educational process. This approach would begin to get more directly at the relationship between lifelong learning and life-span development.[1]

2. The Application of Findings in the Cognitive Area to Research Which Involves Externally Valid Interventions in Meaningful Environments. In order to maximize learning, training in the utilization of effective organizational and mediational strategies should be incorporated into education programs. This should also include research on the fluid intelligence dimension and speed of performance, and possible methodologies for the modification of any apparent decrement. More extensive use of operant techniques in this domain should be investigated and applied to both the human services and lifelong learning context. Furthermore, when considering the heterogeneity in life experiences of all adults, it is necessary to research possible remedial techniques which would be useful in reducing the existing variability in knowledge and learning capabilities.

This area lends itself to some specific demonstrations of technique—in both the lifelong learning and human services contexts. As perhaps its highest single priority it also suggests the necessity of long-term programmatic research to develop measures of external validity.

3. The Development of Research Methodologies That Can Be Utilized Effectively in the Development of Education for Human Services. Typically, human services training programs neglect to link knowledge production with knowledge utilization. Research is needed to link the known methods for effective delivery of human services to educational programs for human service providers. If one wants to assure the most effective training, a compromise between external and internal validity must be worked out. Strict control group designs with random sampling will have to be replaced with quasi-experimental designs which allow for more widespread and less costly training. The potential for use of other methodologies lies relatively untapped in the literature. This is not to say that programs should be haphazardly implemented. Collaborative planning and formulation of objectives between researcher and practitioner should precede such projects. General goals of training such as changes in factual knowledge, skill acquisition, or changes in self-perception and empathic abilities should be objectively measured within the overall framework of improving service delivery systems.

Evaluation research here should not be solely product-oriented nor tied to meeting a deadline for the training of personnel to deliver a mandated service. Let those be the goals of in-service training programs. Rather, the priority here should be given to utilizing good basic research through an educational medium with measurable outcomes and with special emphasis on process variables.[2]

4. The Consideration and Development of Strategies for the Assessment of Educational Outcomes—Both for Human Services Delivery Systems and in Lifelong Learning Contexts. This paper has highlighted—with some dismay—the proliferation of idiosyncratic or charismatic education programs in both contexts. Idiosyncrasy is here defined as programs lacking predictable or at least measurable outcomes.[3] An important role in the area of education research is to provide the leadership for developing and demonstrating strategies for the assessment of educational programs—both for lifelong learning and for human services delivery systems. This implies a dual funding commitment: to methodological development—known to be a slow and tedious process; and, to avoiding the common pitfall of "evaluation hypocrisy" when funding demonstration programs.

Assessment and evaluation contain many facets. One important aspect to be considered is the modification of attitudes of adults towards their own aging process as well as towards other adults as learners and recipients of their services. In addition to this somewhat alleviative direction, a primary preventive approach based on a life-span perspective could be implemented at various age levels. Another area which cannot be dealt with at any length here is the use of demographic data and variables. At this point, rather than specifically gathering extensive new data, we need demonstrations of programs which systematically utilize and check which demographic factors are important to program success. Good evaluation studies here would greatly assist subsequent program planning.

5. *Topical Research Areas.* There are many central issues and topics in this general area today which generate much current discussion on a very anecdotal level. It is recommended that we encourage research and development of many of these ideas on an empirical level through demonstration and exploratory studies. Three of these areas are listed here as examples, although the list is by no means comprehensive. It is not recommended that any one of these topics should become a central research thrust. However, the funding of a few pilot studies in each area could well stimulate and advance the development of more refined researchable hypotheses for future research. In effect, the recommendation here is to promote the state-of-the-art through research of a fairly topical and narrow focus.

a. Research needs to be conducted on *intellectual exercise* independent of learning programs and educational goals. Intellectual exercise of various levels, types, and duration should be studied as a form of human service.

b. Although a great deal is said about the effects of intergenerational interactions, little research to date has suggested ways for modifying and structuring positive intergenerational learning contexts.

c. Research needs to be carried out on the educational counseling process as it affects adults through the life span.

Whereas past program development has been largely divorced from any relevant data base, this paper speaks to the necessity of a research-oriented approach to creating and maintaining educational endeavors in gerontology. Such an approach must be systematic rather than serendipitous. And, in a period where few resources are available for gerontological research and education, much priority must be given to two things: (1) educational programs which will truly facilitate and sustain meaningful adult learning in any context; and (2) the development of educational research methodologies which will provide for objective replications of success and eliminations of failure and overlap.

Finally, at first glance this paper seemed to speak of diverse elements and issues—somewhat loosely organized under the rubric of a research perspective of education in the context of human services and delivery systems. However, it is increasingly evident that future successes in research for both education for human service delivery and lifelong education are closely linked to the application of basic adult learning research and to methodological improvements for applied research.

Notes

1.   For example: Assuming a course in speed-reading is relevant to most people, the purpose and product of such a course contain widely ranging values for different age groups. For the young adult, a speed-reading course might be viewed as a potential boon to assist in the completion of academic assignments. It may provide the middle aged a greater facility for job completion, and hence advancement. In contrast to aiding goal completion, the same course might assist the older adult to understand and expand his knowledge of the world at large at a time when it appears to be shrinking.

2.   The educational application of many years research in the area of age-related sensory impairment is only one recent example of a type of utilization project needed to complete the linkage between the generation-dissemination-utilization-refined generation . . . process (cf. Hickey, 1975b).

3.   It has long been a well-known fact that when many successful programs are subjected to cost-benefit analysis, they are found to be grossly extravagant and not feasible to replicate; yet they are frequently given much play by the field and the media. An equally well-established fact is that many current and recent intergenerational and lifelong learning programs are somewhat serendipitously directed from an anti-research base.

References

Learning and Cognitive Behavior

Baltes, P. Longitudinal and cross-sectional sequences in the study of age and generation effects. *Human Development*, 1968, *11*, 145–171.

Baltes, P., and Labouvie, G. Adult development of intellectual performance: Description, explanation, modification. In C. Eisdorfer and M. Lawton (Eds.), *The psychology of adult development and aging*. Washington, D.C.: American Psychological Association, 1973.

Botwinick, J., and Storandt, M. *Memory, related functions and age*. Springfield, Ill.: Charles C. Thomas, 1974.

Canestrari, R. Age changes in acquisition. In G. G. Talland (Ed.), *Human aging and behavior*. New York: Academic Press, 1968.

Canestrari, R. Paced and self-paced learning in young and elderly adults. *Journal of Gerontology*, 1963, *18*, 165–168.

Cattell, R. B. Theory of fluid and crystallized intelligence: A critical experiment. *Journal of Educational Psychology*, 1963, *54*, 1–22.

Eisdorfer, C. Verbal learning and response time in the aged. *Journal of Genetic Psychology*, 1965, *107*, 15–22.

Eisdorfer, C., Nowlin, J., and Wilkie, F. Improvement of learning in the aged by modification of autonomic nervous system activity. *Science*, 1970, *170*, 1327–1329.

Horn, J., and Cattell, R. Age differences in fluid and crystallized intelligence. *Acta Psychologica*, 1967, *16*(1), 107–129.

Horn, J., and Cattell, R. Age differences in primary mental ability factors. *Journal of Gerontology*, 1966, *21*, 210–220.

Hoyer, W., Labouvie, G., and Baltes, P. Modification of response speed deficits and intellectual performance in the elderly. *Human Development*, 1973, *16*, 233–242.

Hulicka, I. Age differences in retention as a function of interference. *Journal of Gerontology*, 1967, *22*, 180–184.

Hultsch, D. Adult age differences in the organization of free recall. *Developmental Psychology*, 1969, *1*, 673–678.

Hultsch, D. Personal communication, 1975.

Looft, W. Reflections on intervention in old age: Motives, goals and assumptions. *Gerontologist*, 1973, *13*, 6–10.

Monge, R., and Hultsch, D. Paired-associate learning as a function of adult age and the length of the anticipation and inspection levels. *Journal of Gerontology*, 1971, *26*, 157–162.

Plemons, J., Willis, S., and Baltes, P. Challenging the theory of fluid intelligence: A training approach. Paper presented at 28th Meeting Gerontological Society, Louisville, Kentucky, October 1975.

Powell, A., Eisdorfer, C., and Bogdonoff, M. Physiologic response patterns observed in a learning task. *Archives of General Psychiatry*, 1964, *10*, 192–195.

Schaie, K. A general model for the study of developmental problems. *Psychological Bulletin*, 1965, *64*, 92–107.

Woodruff, D., and Birren, J. Biofeedback conditioning of the EEG alpha rhythm in young and old subjects. *Proceedings of the 80th Annual Meeting of the American Psychological Association*, Honolulu, Hawaii, 1972.

Woodruff, D., and Walsh, D. Research in adult learning: The individual. *Gerontologist*, 1975, *15* (5), 424–430.

Adult Education

Boyle, P., and Jahns, I. Program development and evaluation. In R. Smith, G. Aker, and J. Kidd (Eds.), *Handbook of adult education*. New York: Macmillan, 1970.

Hesburgh, T., Miller, P., and Wharton, C. *Patterns of lifelong learning*. San Francisco: Jossey-Bass, 1973.

Houle, C. *The design of education*. San Francisco: Jossey-Bass, 1973.

Scully, M. Carnegie Commission asks colleges to alter admissions patterns, take more adults, transfers. *Chronicle of Higher Education,* August 27, 1973, 7.

Smith, R., Aker, G., and Kidd, J. (Eds.). *Handbook of adult education.* New York: Macmillan, 1970.

Education for Human Services and Applied Training

Connelly, J. A model for organization and evaluation of short-term training. *Gerontologist,* 1975, *15* (5), 442–447.

Hickey, T. Continuing education in gerontology for allied health. *Journal of Allied Health,* 1975a, *4*(3), 5–12.

Hickey, T. Simulating age-related sensory impairments for practitioner education. *Gerontologist,* 1975b, *15* (5), 457–463.

Zerbe, M., and Hickey, T. Self-maintenance skills for geriatric nursing. *Journal of Gerontological Nursing,* May/June 1975, *1* (2), 5–9.

Miscellaneous

Chiles, L. *Training needs in gerontology.* Hearings before the U.S. Senate Special Committee on Aging, June 19, 1973. Washington, D. C.: U. S. Government Printing Office.

White House Conference on Aging. *Toward a national policy on aging.* Proceedings, Vol. II, 1971.

Section Two

Major Issues:
Future Directions

The author of the first paper in this section expresses his view of major issues and trends in academic gerontology. The following two articles are responses to his presentation. The reader will recognize the persistence of certain themes and concerns and various perspectives concerning the themes and concerns running through all of the articles in Section Two.

Great Issues in Academic Gerontology: Where Are We Going and Why?

K. Warner Schaie
University of Southern California

It is a great pleasure to be able to talk about future directions in gerontology today because, when I got my doctoral degree (doing a dissertation which today would probably be described as a gerontological one), there weren't any jobs for gerontologists. And in fact people viewed my interest in aging out of the corner of the eye as if they thought I was talking about something a little weird. The implication was: Why don't you do something mainline? Why do you engage in something which, if you really understood the system, will only be a career hazard to you? I feel that we have reached the stage where gerontology, if it isn't mainline, is well on the way to becoming mainline, and where several of the major disciplines that saw the influx of aging as a sort of maverick at the outset are now very pleased to find that their institution has somebody in the discipline who knows something about aging.

I think we have come of age, and yet I'm a little concerned about the notion of great issues—who knows what great issues are? But there are many issues in academic gerontology, and I will try to do about the only thing that I can do with the task that I have been assigned: That is, I shall essentially give my very personalized associations to what seem to me some of the salient issues that academicians in gerontology are facing or should be facing today and perhaps raise some cautions for those of you who are relatively new in the field from one who can almost take a historical perspective on how academia has very slowly backed into the field of gerontology, and how this causes a real hazard to us.

Frequently, when one has lived this sort of thing, one has the feeling that a person coming in new might see it in a much more constructive manner. Very often we old timers tend to protract and perpetuate the problems of yesterday—the problems that we know—while those who are new in the field are talking about the problems of tomorrow. Nevertheless, I think that there is much truth to the adage that if one doesn't understand one's history one is destined to repeat it and this adage probably holds for gerontology as for any other socially responsible field.

There are three broad areas where one might make some appropriate comments. I would like to subdivide my talk into issues related to *manpower development*, issues related to *training*, and issues related to *substance*. This may be a peculiar ordering of priorities, but it is a necessary one because the substantive issues in gerontology are innumerable. Our ability to deal with them effectively is directly related to the question: Can we produce well-trained individuals? How do we train individuals to attack issues, in particular, the issue of where the manpower is going to come from? Some years ago, I gave a paper at the Gerontological Society called "Training the Trainers of Trainers." And that's where we essentially still are, because we find ourselves suddenly called upon to develop a large pool of manpower in the service provider areas and the assumption is made that if we only had the money to fund these efforts we could do it.

Now the fact is that a group as large as the one attending this meeting creates the implication that there is enough institutional interest and ability to use substantial training funds if they were provided. But that's a very false notion. What would we do if we were to receive a large sum of money; if some benevolent deity were to drop all the money in the world upon us? How would we deal with this in an orderly fashion?

And so I must make the statement—in spite of the number of people here today, in spite of the enormous contributions of such organizations as the Gerontological Society and many other professional groups, we still do not have an adequate cadre of trainers. We still find that the same people appear on all the programs wherever you go. We still find that it's a buddy-buddy system. And the reason for this state of affairs is really very simple—the number of people who indeed have a sufficient commitment, who are willing to undertake serious training tasks within the academic process, is severely limited. In fact one might argue that at the present time there are probably no more than six or eight programs or centers in this country that could efficiently utilize substantial amounts of new training funds, programs which would not be restricted to two- or three-day workshops for this, that, or the other group, but would use the money for the purpose of training professionals whose lifetime vocation would indeed be the teaching and training of people in the various disciplines that come together to form what we call gerontology. We still have the problem that we have only a small number of institutions that could even begin to expand the training of this cadre. That's how our problem begins.

Now a second problem is that, if you happen to be associated with one of the currently active programs, everyone thinks this way of thinking is nonsense, that what I am really talking about is a guild issue. I may be asked whether I am not simply trying to protect my own program? I say this is nonsense. Suppose we were to declare open season and proceed to raid the faculty of existing programs. Let us even assume for the moment that everybody in the business who has had experience developing programs at the graduate level, who could get those people trained who are going to work at training, people who have a long-term academic commitment—if everyone in this field would be available on the job market, we still wouldn't have the capability of providing each one of your institutions with a senior gerontologist to start a new program. All we would be doing is commercializing the existing centers, to open up new centers in other locations, and we would be playing no more than a game of musical chairs.

A related manpower issue I would like to raise is the problem that those of you who are in the process of developing new centers are going to adversely affect the development and expansion of the manpower cadre, the training cadre, if you raid existing programs of their senior people because all you would be doing is moving a training site from one institution to another. I would strongly urge those institutions that are developing training programs at the graduate level to consider two things: First, identify the senior individuals on your staff who are going to enter the field of gerontology—that is, people who are experienced academic administrators—and allow them the opportunities to go to existing centers as visiting scientists and let them have the opportunity to develop some substantive expertise in their field related to gerontology; second, if you must raid other institutions, do so at the level of more junior people, who in order of their own career progressions logically should be the core faculty of other developing institutions.

Again, this may be a very selfish position, but I think it is not as selfish as it might seem because one of the things that I am very much concerned about is the fact that not only do I find it very difficult to train a substantial number of these cadre individuals in our own center, but I don't see very many eligible candidates when I recount each year to fill one or two openings that might develop as we expand. We all have the responsibility, if we are thinking of a serious, high quality development in academic gerontology, to pay a lot more attention to cadre-building than we have done in the past.

Now, what are some of the manpower demands we have to be concerned about? Thus far, I have discussed the issues related to the provision of a basic cadre. But, let me go one step further; obviously we must train individuals for community and four-year college. It is very likely that one of the great breakthroughs in the field of gerontology will occur when we make an impact at the level of mass education. That is the point where we might gain access to the educators who do not necessarily go all the way around graduate programs, but who are found in the liberal arts and professional education programs. I think one of the essential issues is whether or not we can be sure that the manpower pool we start will have in it most of the basic disciplines dealing with human services and understanding of human problems—people concerned with gerontology. We should make sure that every four-year college has at least one sociologist, one psychologist, one biologist, one economist, who, because of background and training, has a commitment to gerontology, would see it as natural, that it's not just a matter of teaching such a person a course in the biology of aging, but that the issue is: Would a biologist teaching an introductory biology course find it necessary and essential to address issues of aging? And it seems to me that this kind of manpower development is not just a matter of training specialists but of training people who are going to see gerontological issues as essential to their particular disciplinary offerings.

The third area, of course, is the issue of mental health specialists. A recent manpower report on aging and mental health confronts us with statistics that about better than a quarter of services for mental health go to the elderly, while less than one percent of the available manpower has been prepared for services to the elderly. And again we find ourselves in a catch-22 position. I was asked to do a position paper related to the problems in developing a manpower pool in clinical psychology. Well, when I started playing the numbers game, and I simply counted how many people we have now who can train clinical psychologists interested in aging, it turned out that the minimal time plan required to obtain trained people who would generate the projected manpower, would be a ten-year program—one which is going to involve very careful planning because it would have to start out with the very few programs that would train people who could then develop new programs. We discovered that if we were to develop immediately a whole bunch of new programs, we would first have to declare a moratorium on psychological services to the elderly because we would have to offer academic employment to every single individual who has been identified as having an interest in the elderly. I looked at some of the other position papers and what I have said about psychology is equally true in social work, more true in nursing, and so down the line.

The fourth area where I find high needs for manpower development is the issue of program evaluation specialist. We find that, of necessity in any emerging field when funds are available to staff organizations such as the Area Agencies on Aging, it is necessary to invite staff who have had no previous association with the field of aging, but who have some kind of administrative skill and some kind of involvement in delivery of services.

Now we find that as a consequence, the issue of evaluation of programs is a lot more critical because of a real paradox: Some of these people obviously are doing all sorts of wrong things, but also some are by sheer luck or favorable circumstances doing a lot of right things. And it behooves us to find out.

Again, we have a serious lack in terms of manpower involved in program evaluation; we are beginning to get quite a bit of theoretical formulation. But there is really no adequate manpower available that could be applied to monitor the many programs which are now emerging.

And finally in the area of manpower, I would like to call attention to the great need for the development of academic training programs for what we might call program development specialists. Again, one of the big issues we face is that in the area of aging, it is not simply a matter of extending available programming to a new population. Rather, it's a matter of dealing with the issue that as a society we really have very little experience in understanding what might be meaningful alternatives, meaningful life roles for the elderly. And here we have grounds for developing a new breed of individuals, who are able to address these issues rather than let things happen, because we are beginning to generate a limited knowledge. While it doesn't really tell us what to do, it certainly tells us what are some of the things to avoid and some of the directions in which we might move.

I mentioned some of the manpower issues; let me expand a little on the training issues. First, how do we deal with the immediate pressures? The academic community is in a much better position to resist the event of instant gerontology than other sectors of society are. As we all know, often to our chagrin, academic systems move very slowly. Sometimes this may not be all bad, because it seems to me that while we obviously do not wish to declare a moratorium, we do have to insist that we have a time frame within which we can move. Academic inertia may, in fact, be helpful in providing us with a time frame that permits some orderly development.

I think that such orderly development requires two stages. At most institutions, it will require a very substantial effort to infiltrate some of the existing disciplines. We are all very much aware that while most universities and colleges are making this effort (and that is why we have such a large group of people at this meeting), we can typically identify no more than one or two individuals who are interested in issues of aging or who have even done some work or teaching in this area. But what we typically do not have is a situation where any one institution clearly has been infiltrated in terms of all of the disciplines that one would like to have address the issues of aging. And so one of the first steps an institution should address is the procedure of infiltration.

It may be that a sound investment of initial institutional resources would be to provide career incentives by rewarding individuals in the core disciplines of universities for spending some of their time, for moving more strongly in the area of aging, or for considering aging as a worthwhile endeavor. Here are a number of mechanisms that can be applied. There have been a number of workshops for faculty conducted by one or two institutions. The Gerontological Society used to have a program of that kind. It is hoped that we will move in that area again in the near future. But it seems to me that, if an institution is really serious in mounting an effort in gerontology, a good expenditure of institutional resources would indeed be to supply some limited resources to encourage faculty, critically selected faculty in various areas, to attend some of these seminars and thereby increase the nucleus of interested people in an institution. I think that it may be well worthwhile to increase the opportunities for established individuals who might wish to move into the area of gerontology to develop such skills without making it a particular career hazard, and without it requiring a significant financial investment on their part.

I hope, at some point, we can convince funding agencies that it may be well worthwhile to provide more support for the visiting scientist model because one of the ways in which cadres could be substantially increased at a relatively limited cost is for the existing centers that do have a quantum of gerontology-related interests to host visitors from other institutions. This depends, of course, on finding a mechanism that would encourage individuals to come and to look upon this as a career enhancement.

As we go into training, we obviously are going to have to face a whole slew of difficult issues. I am well aware of some of the concerns of this group, as well as of the Gerontological Society, about the issue of credentials, and of maintenance of standards, and I think that these efforts are very worthwhile. But I think we are going to be emasculated, or perhaps we will even fail, if we do not take into account the guild interests of the established professions. It seems to me that we will have to step very carefully in this matter because, at the level of the professions and the academic institutions, you get tremendous resentment if you tell these people what they should do and what curriculum they should have. We will have to work very closely with the existing professions. These are not insurmountable issues, but I think they are ones that those of us concerned with training are going to have to pay very close attention to. Obviously, it would be irresponsible if we were to train individuals who would be promptly shut out because we have not protected our potential trainees from the realities of professional organization and professional guild issues.

Now some other issues that seem to me important are that we ought to have some very clear models in academia about what it is that we are training for. As you know, the Andrus Gerontology Center has gone with a vengeance into the business of granting professional degrees in gerontology. I do not know whether it really makes sense to provide these people with research training. My feeling is that the service provider ought to be trained to be a reasonably competent research consumer. In other words, if you are a service provider, you ought to be able to read a research article and speculate what it might mean for your particular application. But I don't really think it's profitable and very likely to increase our knowledge base if we insist on building research competence into a brief masters program which will be to train service providers. Those of us who edited the recent series of handbooks in basic research in gerontology were impressed by the tremendous increase of information, but depressed by the tremendous amount of blind alleys that people have gone into. There is a tremendous amount of research that suggests very exciting possibilities, but when you read the fine print the work remains exciting only if you are going to ignore issues such as reliability or validity of instruments or if you are going to ignore often miniscule sample sizes. So, we have a lot of knowledge, but it's not a very deep knowledge base. And I'm deathly afraid of the possibility that the mass training implementation will not be at the doctoral level but will be at the bachelor's and master's level. All these people are going to be expected to do publishable master's theses. I shudder at the amount of misdirection that the field may receive by very well meaning young and not-so-young people who are being taught by academic institutions to do things which are not really appropriate to their career objectives.

Another thing we have to worry about is that we may have little opportunity to experiment with modern models of training. We should not get tied up in saying let's continue business as usual, with the established training models. An exciting aspect of gerontology is that, more than any other field, it is very likely to have a true life-span clientele. That is, gerontology is going to be the field of the mature learner; and one of the things we have to worry about is that we know as gerontologists that middle-aged and old people don't learn in the same way that twenty-year-olds do; and I think some of our training programs are going to have to be at the forefront of showing how one educates adults.

In one sense, this is perhaps one of the great academic issues in gerontology. Can we, at least while we are training gerontologists, provide a training model that will demonstrate what the education of mature and older people is going to be like in comparison to education of young adults? This does not necessarily mean that we are going to be entirely different. There may be opportunities for accelerated training when we are working with a clientele who may have a great deal more life experience than most younger people do. It may even be that an extended schedule of training is needed when we are training older individuals in specific skills. We know that training middle-aged and older persons requires a different type of patience. But I think that here we have some great opportunities to influence academic systems because one of the things we know is that in terms of the change in the demographic structure of society most academic institutions and particularly the broad-based institutions, such as the community college, are going to be in great trouble if they continue to see the young as their primary clientele. I think as academic gerontologists, we can help institutions to go through this transition. In many institutions this development is already upon us and we are coping with it. But it is going to come upon all of us whether as academicians we like it or not.

I would now like to mention a number of substantive issues. After all, academia is not just supposed to be form, academia is supposed to be substance as well. We are the people who dream of the future. We may not always be successful, but we make the glorious attempt to move society into what we think is a more humane direction, a more just direction. We may fall down on all these counts, but when we don't think of budget, these are some of the things that we perhaps do pay some attention to. I might argue that at the level of influencing society, of generating new knowledge bases, it is obviously impossible for any one institution to cover the entire field. It might behoove any emerging group to think about what the particular area is and where it wishes to make its impact. It is obvious that there are some issues that cut across fields and that may well deserve serious attention by some institutions. There are indeed broad areas for interdisciplinary areas that may be useful.

In regards to biological science, I would like to say that one of the major educational enterprises one must be concerned with in academia is to provide some understanding that the issue is not merely the search for life prolongation. We need to concern ourselves with creating an understanding that even if there were some major breakthrough on life prolongation issues, these issues may more likely affect the lives of our grandchildren and great-grandchildren. One of the more basic concerns is a better understanding of the control mechanisms which would lead not to life prolongation, but to an increase in the quality of life. Those of us concerned with learning processes of the older individual are very much aware of the fact that biological scientists could help us in our understanding of what is going on in the aging nervous system. Often, when we think we have taught an older person something, we really haven't, because the aging nervous system just wasn't alert when we were there. We might then be able to engage in very substantial break-throughs in dealing with what may not be intellectual decrement but is due to behavioral obsolescence. We've got to deal with the fact that the elderly nervous system is the control mechanism involved here, and we need a better understanding. Very likely, if we understand the control mechanisms, we could do remarkable things to increase the quality of life for individuals. We want to make sure that if, indeed, we should live longer, there is some point to it.

In the behavioral sciences, one of the priority issues that I think we are going to have to address is what some people call functional age. One of the exciting things about adults' behavior is that there is so much more plasticity there than in the behavior of children. The range of adaptive behavior in children is very limited, but in adults is virtually unlimited.

Certainly, at some point, in the not-so-distant future, somebody is going to tell us that discrimination by age is just as bad as discrimination by ethnic group, or sex, and when that comes about, gerontologists will be faced with the problem of providing a knowledge base other than chronological age to retire people. And before we can do this, we had better understand the full complexity of the issues. To give an example, a favorite stereotype of psychologists is the notion that when young people fail in a task it is because of an error of commission while old people make errors of omission. We have recently shown that this information has nothing to do with age, but is related to the nature of the task. In the behavioral sciences we are still at a very basic level in gerontology when it comes to understanding some of the complex phenomena. We certainly have only begun to look at issues such as cross-ethnic variations in aging.

Some other issues: Why is it that some people are treated as if they were old when they are in their forties and other people are treated as if they had never heard the word aging when they are quite elderly? I have the feeling that here we are not talking about the issue of aging, but of the notion of power and powerlessness. But some of these issues need more attention. And of course, there is the impact of the changing population structure in the future, because it is quite clear that those of us who have looked at old people for some time know that the aged of 20 years hence will be quite different from those of today.

And there's one thing that gerontologists often forget that they have going for them. If you are going to predict what children will be like who are born 50 years from now, you are in very bad shape because it will be 50 years before they are born. Now, for the gerontologist, everyone who will turn 65 years old for the next 65 years has already been born—at least you know their number—but there are many other variables which we know can help us predict trends later, directionally.

On the issue of environment, I think that we have not yet really looked at the implications of age integration and age segregation, or of the environmental impact of legislation which may make segregation more difficult even when desirable, communal living arrangements for the elderly. We have all these ordinances that are designed to keep the hippies out of the community, but also make it impossible to develop suitable housing alternatives for the elderly. Another important issue is the lack of spatial arrangements which compensate for perceptual loss. It turns out that one of the biggest problems that old people have in the urban environment is the fact that the architecture of buildings is typically designed for the young. The aging nervous system requires greater distances between signs than what would be perceived by a 35-year-old traffic engineer. There are obviously a number of environmental issues around which gerontological research could be built.

Let me address the issue of health services. One of my real fears, now that the first American chair of Geriatrics has been endowed and filled, is that medicine is going to discover a new disease called "aging." It seems to me that certainly the phenomenon of aging is a psychosocial and biological phenomenon, which obviously has many implications for medicine but is not basically a problem of illness. In fact, I would argue that delivery of health services for the elderly would become much more manageable if we were dealing with issues of preventive health care for the elderly—coming back to the issue of longevity. We have created an environment in which the infant can survive. Some of this involves medical care, but more of it involves adequate education. Mothers do not kill their young infants anymore as they used to by exposing them to unnecessary environmental hazards. I think we still allow a great many adults to kill themselves by inadequate preventive health care. What we need is a broad concern in how we can maintain the health of our elderly population.

I could have covered all sorts of other issues, but I think I covered the critical ones in academic gerontology today.

Commentary

Charles Gaitz
Texas Research Institute of Mental Sciences

I do not consider myself to be truly academia, and it is from the vantage point of a practitioner that I will make my remarks. I had neither seen nor heard Warner's paper until now. It seems to me that the great issues in academic gerontology hinge upon a very fundamental question—Who is a gerontologist? Maybe you know, but when you come to me and my medical colleagues, we often do not know about whom you are talking.

If we identify you as a social gerontologist, this begins to narrow things a little bit. But the critical issue, it seems to me, is to identify who is the gerontologist and how that person becomes one. Is it by experience? Is it by training? Or is it by education? What are the qualifications? I would also ask you to make up your minds whether gerontology should be a term synonymous with social gerontology.

Maybe there is a need for other modifiers. Maybe we need terms like child gerontology, medical gerontology, psychiatric gerontology. At one level, you might think that ridiculous, but it seems to me to be a very fundamental question to address.

What is social gerontology? Is it analogous to what might be a part of a personality development course for medical students? Is it an essential basic science for anthropologists and psychologists in the sense that anatomy, physiology, or pharmacology might be basic sciences for students of medicine? Should social gerontology be a designation for special emphasis in a discipline such as psychology? In my judgment, all of these and similar questions are critical ones because of the ease with which one becomes identified as an expert.

You must not knock the notion of instant gerontologists. Most of us in medicine who are identified with aging have had little or no formal training in geriatric medicine. Speaking for myself, after a number of years in practice, I decided to find out what academia was like by jumping in and doing something in a department of psychiatry. I became the director of residency training. My qualifications for the position were primarily that I had been a psychiatrist for a while and I was interested in teaching. The department of psychiatry needed somebody to coordinate its residency training program. I spent three years in this capacity. By then I was an "expert" in residency training. A number of other psychiatrists joined the department and did not have specific jobs. Because I had been a consultant at a home for the aged, that "qualified" me as a specialist in geriatric psychiatry. And someone else became the "expert" in residency training. That's the way the world is. A few weeks ago I spoke with a child psychiatrist who is now 52. He expressed an interest in gerontology. I told him he too could become an expert in geriatric psychiatry relatively easily. Now obviously I am here today not because I am an expert in social gerontology but because I am the president of the Gerontological Society and *should* know and do certain things. I spoke a few weeks ago with people from mental health centers about programs for the aged. If you just accept these people as being kind, gentle, well-motivated, you can sometimes get them interested in aging. But if you set up rigid standards and you say, "If you're going to work with older people, you have to know more about yourself and have special training," what really happens is that they're not only scared away from getting involved, but they use the lack of knowledge as a cop-out. They have a good excuse to explain why they are not going to take care of old people. They minimize what they already know as trained persons. Experts telling us we have to know a great deal about gerontology before getting started may actually inhibit program development. This is why I emphasize the definition of the role of gerontologist.

Today, meeting with gerontologists, I talk the language of gerontology, while last week I was talking the language of psychiatry because I was at a meeting of psychiatrists. The issues, the problems, are not at all different. We talked about problems of role identification for psychiatrists just as today we are concerned with role identification for gerontologists. There are all sorts of ways to be a gerontologist or a psychiatrist. To illustrate this point, let us recall what a psychiatrist does and what the responsibility is. We are going through a period in which primary-care physicians will be doing what psychiatrists have been doing. Consequently, this means that there will have to be changes in role and clarification of what a psychiatrist will do in the future, and this will affect standards and training.

Whether we are thinking of gerontology and gerontologists or psychiatry and psychiatrists, setting up standards and licensing practitioners doesn't solve all the problems. Constant monitoring and changes are necessary.

There are some disadvantages to being certified. Let us look into the matter of continuing education. Obviously, it is "good." But continuing education under what conditions? What should be the content? Why should only the "certified" specialists be required to obtain continuing education? There are gerontologists working at mental health centers, there are gerontologists working at universities, and gerontologists working in research labs. Obviously the standards and requirements for continuing education are going to be far different. Furthermore, even if you set up a system of certification, you'll find out that not everyone needs to be certified to get a particular job. An uncertified person can obtain a job making twice as much money as a certified specialist; certification may not be important to an employer. Yet, in order to be recertified, the specialists will have to be reexamined to be recertified! And the uncertified person goes on doing, working, being paid without these burdens of continuing education, recertification, etc. We want higher standards in places where they are needed, but certification and training standards are only part of what will achieve this goal.

Commentary

George Maddox
Duke University

I was in an airplane all last night in getting here, and this morning I was looking at the ceiling and someone said, "Are you sure you know where you are?" I'm not sure I know where I am, but I do want to indicate that it's been a pleasure to hear Warner. I recall days when we were on a study section together at NIH. We used to have conversations, and the issues haven't changed over the years.

Warner has made many points. When you reflect on the notes you've taken, you will find that you have, in fact, been exposed to a dramatic discussion on those fundamental issues that have been around for awhile and are going to be around for awhile.

First, what's in a name? This may say something about our newness in some sense in that we worry about who we are and what we are supposed to be doing. I'm not sure myself how important the selection of a label should be. It may be that we should be able to learn to live with different labels, and I've been doing that for a long time. I hear people say, "Are you a gerontologist?" and I say, "Certainly." And they say, "Are you attached to that term?" and I say, "No." I find that when I talk to different people I use different words. When I use the term gerontology, they always get defensive with me. I think we need to concentrate on what our issues are and what we think we are doing. And we should worry about the guild-like issues and the labels we should use. I don't believe this is unimportant. I think that the issues in gerontology for the next decade will depend on what we choose to label ourselves.

Second, I want to suggest that learning to live with the implications of specialization, which is something that all American professionals have had to struggle with for a long time, is something we will continue to struggle with in the future. We have segmented ourselves to death. That area we call human aging or gerontology has not been exempt from this problem nor will we be exempt from it. What I have enjoyed and appreciated as an academic and professional working in this area is that I think my colleagues worry about the issue of the fragmentation and worry about how they can minimize it more than any other collection of professionals with whom I've identified. I think those who belong to the community that we'll call, for convenience, gerontology, worry more about the problems of this society and about how professionals are going to relate to it more effectively than most of my other colleagues. For example, as a member of the National Institute on Aging Council, I find that Council worrying more than the average council about these issues. I think that this sophist society, AGHE, or the Geriatric Society, or the Gerontological Society, has taken on the major problem of this society, and I'm pleased to be a part of addressing that issue.

Another issue Warner spoke of is the problem of this organization and organizations such as Area Agencies on Aging and the Commission on Aging. The problem is that those who work with this community called aging do not speak with the same voice and this doesn't surprise me. But, we come here talking about academics and the support of academia. Recently we had a meeting in which a group of people said, "Academics need to recognize their responsibility of translating what they are doing to the 'using' community out there." And somebody said, "Let's hear it for that." Now someone says, "Let's hear it from the user community." It is our responsibility to make sure that academicians are strong in order that there can be a basis for the exchange. I think that gerontologists worry about that issue more than most do. It's not just the matter of believing that academe has nothing to offer. Academe must translate what it knows so that the knowledge can be used. At the same time, the consumer has to indicate the belief that it is important to have a strong academic institution working in this area.

Let me shift the emphasis to manpower. Warner, as he starts counting noses of people calling themselves gerontologists, sees a lack of time, especially in terms of what he calls cadres. We need to put back into context with our awareness the fact that there is increasingly a very large pool of highly trained manpower. I do not know a labor economist who does not say that we have a problem on our hands. We have too large a pool of highly trained manpower at the present time. The question clearly then is not the absence of the manpower, it is that their specialty training does not match well with where manpower is needed.

There are two implications, both of them interesting and one of them rather disturbing. One is that with the large existing manpower pool, we need to be talking about retreading people and reorienting their training. If we could do this, we could meet many of our manpower problems in gerontology without training a single new person. And we could do it for a long period of time. That's on the one hand. On the other hand, given what we know about the need of maintaining the vitality of disciplines, of introducing new and innovative ideas, we simply cannot stand where we are. This is one of the great problems currently being addressed by academes, not just gerontologists, but all universities. As you know, we are just now around 80 percent of the people in institutions who are tenured. With the possibility of a few pushes and pulls here and there, we might have 100 percent tenured faculty in a short period of time, with no jobs for young faculty. That's the worst scenario. As a matter of fact, in gerontology we need to recognize that there is a large pool of people for whom retreading is one of our options. I hope that as we talk about these issues we will lead new people into this particular field.

Warner was talking about various ways in which we might address the issues. Some of these have to do with retreading and trying to maintain the interest of people already working. This is sometimes called add-ons. For example, we talked about visiting scientists. I have had on my mind in recent years, the need to have something like a board in the medical field for behavioral and social scientists. Speaking of career development in existing institutions, for example, I was pleased that my institution recently provided money for career development awards for new faculty in gerontology. These did not start with predoctoral students, but were for established junior scientists who can now compete for career development awards internally through our institution. I am aware that the Gerontological Society has had a different approach. We pay scientists to come and visit communities. It is really rather curious that gerontology is interested in services delivered because we are bringing service-delivery people to the institutions who say, "Let us tell you what we know."

Another educational issue that Warner spoke of and that I also want to underline is that because we call ourselves gerontologists it does not mean that we know everything we need to know about working with older people or about training. One of the things that impressed me is the applicability of an old saw that war is too important a business to be left to generals. Gerontology, in terms of its multifacets, may be too important to be left to gerontologists. Let me give you some illustrations.

If in my institution we work on issues of training, I would discover that when I want to turn to a person who knows something about education or learning technology, I don't usually find that the person I turn to is a gerontologist. People who know most, in my experience, about teaching and learning, don't have labels. And I don't think that matters. I think it is critical that gerontology has the advantage of the best learning technology available. I don't want to let the guild issue tell me where I should turn to find that expertise. In the same way, I find that I do not turn to gerontologists to tell me how to organize a service system. I do not think that being a gerontologist necessarily means that you know how to organize service systems.

I do not think that being a gerontologist necessarily tells us whether or not we will have reliable and valid schools to do the kind of research we need to do. This is an important point—What is so exciting to me about the Gerontological Society is the recognition that it has some societally, scientifically, and academically important issues that cannot be reduced to a simple guild issue. That is a problem on which I think the Gerontological Society has worked more carefully and longer than any society that I know about. I think that it is important to work on these issues because everyone who works in the gerontological area and works with older people comes to this recognition. You almost never see a presentation of any problem (i.e., practical service problem, an academic issue). A problem is almost never presented in the simple way that is reducible in anybody's guild. This is one of the things that makes me say that we owe a great debt in this society to older people and to those who have tried to respond to the issues that make life great. I think older people have challenged the society to recognize that both our institutional arrangements and our knowledge base are inadequate. They presented a real challenge.

What is interesting to me in terms of the academic community's response to this is the recognition of the importance and necessity of interdisciplinary response. You cannot deal with issues presented by late life in terms of anybody's guild. You can't reduce them to that. This has resulted in some very stimulating interdisciplinary work in training characteristic of this particular field so that when people ask me, "Do you identify with gerontology?" I say, "Yes, I do." Because not only do I think we have an opportunity to learn something from what's happening in gerontology, I think gerontology has the chance to teach disciplines, something that is very important about the essentials of an interdisciplinary response. I'm enthusiastic about this; so when you ask me, "Are you a gerontologist?" I not only say, "yes," I say, "I'm proud of it."

PART THREE
INFORMAL COMMENTARIES
AND EXPLORATIONS

Section One
Functions of Academic Gerontology and Issues in Program Development

Those teaching courses that have direct, obvious social implications are more concerned with the purpose of their courses than those teaching in other areas. This seems to be particularly true in the earlier developmental stages of an academic discipline. For this reason, gerontology teachers, researchers, and administrators are concerned with the functions of their courses and programs.

Other issues of concern focus on different approaches in teaching gerontology and developing gerontology programs. Educators who want to develop educational programs in gerontology face numerous questions and alternatives. Many of these approaches have been successful; yet each author who describes an approach emphasizes that the individual educational institution must develop its own unique approach to program design. This section reviews issues that must be confronted by anyone developing a new program or expanding an existing involvement.

Functions of Academic Gerontology
(Undergraduate Level)

Cyprian J. Cooney
Mercyhurst College

In talking about the functions of academic gerontology, I am taking the perspective of a credentialed social gerontologist, trained and practised in the "generalist" tradition and engaged as a full-time educator in undergraduate teaching since 1974. I will focus on three of the many aspects of the topic, the functions of academic gerontology.

The first aspect relates to the future functions of academic gerontology. I begin with the future because there seems to be an emerging consensus about the role of academic gerontology. This budding consensus gives me hope. Above all, it gives me, as a representative of undergraduate gerontology, a sense of direction.

There was an analogous consensus among the first generation of academic gerontologists in the 1950s (Donahue, 1960; Koller, 1962; Tibbits, 1960). But, their legacy was dissipated (or did we lose sight of it?) during the ensuing 20 years. In its place there erupted the "blessed chaos" of the early 1970s, which Seltzer described (1974), and which still prevails widely. I will return to this later.

My position is consistent with that of Spinetta and Hickey (1975), Weg (1975), Freeman (1976), Bolton (1976), and others. I believe that academic gerontology is "potentiated" to play a progressively more prominent role on all levels of higher academic activity. Its role will have at least two principal facets. One is concerned with the facilitation of appropriate age-related institutional adjustments. The other focuses upon the identification and communication/integration of human values specific to later life.

In higher education of the future, it will be normal to find a mix of older and young students in most classes. Gerontological sophistication will be a standard criterion of faculty performance. This sophistication will be defined in terms of age awareness, gerontological knowledge, and androgynous techniques. On the administrative level, life-span relevance and effectiveness will determine the design, staffing, and evaluation of programs. Other accommodations related to learning environments, materials, and student credentialing will also be routinized.

In order to facilitate the evolution of those institutional changes, educational consultation will become a more typical professional activity for both resident and visiting academic gerontologists. Correlatively, it will be expected that academic gerontologists will have expertise in the broad technical aspects of life-span education.

On the more substantive level of identifying and communicating/integrating age-related human values, academic gerontology will perform a unique and indispensable function. All of the so-called humanities will be gerontologized in the future. Even philosophy and theology will eventually come into their own as bona fide, developed components of a truly comprehensive, integrated academic gerontology. Ultimately, every academic discipline will feature a focused and articulated gerontological dimension.

During the transition to that stage of development, those physical and social sciences which pioneered the gerontological movement since World War II will serve as much-in-demand models. Their scientists will be primary advocates of this transition. They will be its architects and counselors. The process itself, however, will be dominated by students, young and old. Their value-concerns will energize the process. Their respective, complementary age-related value-postures will supply both substance and direction to the process. The urgency of the future toward the definition and integration of age-related human values will simultaneously break down and reestablish the "territoriality" of each academic discipline, even of those thought to be interdisciplinary. A new role and synthesis for the separate and related activities of all academic disciplines will take shape.

In that context, the AGHE which clings exclusively to an organized concern for gerontology in *higher* education will be progressively divested of a leadership position by an AGE organization, a new association committed to the representation, advocacy, and counseling of life-span gerontology on *all* levels of education. The latter association, by virtue of its vision and plan for hosting/stimulating age awareness, personal development, and intergenerational interaction at each period of the life span, will inspire and direct the ultimate blossoming of academic gerontology.

The second aspect of the "Functions of Academic Gerontology" concerns the present. As coordinator of an undergraduate program of studies on aging, I find myself repeatedly having to face the question: What primary function(s) is academic gerontology supposed to have on the undergraduate level? There are two things about this question that are tormenting. The first is that until now, I have been unable to find an answer to this question—either in the literature, in AGHE, or in myself. The second torment is that until the question is answered, undergraduate academic gerontology will lack direction and, at best, will have provisional rather than stable purpose(s).

Seltzer (1974) has suggested that allowing oneself to be tormented in this context is wasteful of time and energy because the question can neither be asked nor answered along universal or absolute lines. Her position is that undergraduate academic gerontology is essentially a relative entity that can be programmed by each institution in its own particular way. I wish I were more consoled by her approach, since Seltzer is among the very few voices who have addressed this particular issue. Unfortunately, the drummer I hear has yet to be muffled. I have found little consolation and even less insight for my purposes in Seltzer's benediction of the programmatic chaos characterizing much of undergraduate academic gerontology. In my mind, the question still persists. What is/are the primary function(s) of academic gerontology on the undergraduate level? More specifically, do you program undergraduate gerontology as preliminary to future graduate studies? Or, do you program it for baccalaureate-level entry into direct service jobs? Perhaps you program it simply for the stimulation of age awareness in students.

The question has still other dimensions. Do you program undergraduate gerontology as a major course of studies and do you name that major gerontology? Or, do you accommodate your program to the misgivings even of some gerontologists, structuring it as a second major or as a minor, and employing the nomenclature of the related discipline? More problematical yet—do you tilt gerontology on the undergraduate level toward theoretical or applied emphasis? And, do you stress normative aging, developmental or therapeutic gerontology? Do you program requirements, including prerequisites and cognate courses, or merely electives? Do you administer your program within a single discipline or via an interdisciplinary structure of some kind?

Perhaps one does two or more of those things. Perhaps you do as many as you can. Maybe you begin with a course or two and just let things evolve— whatever will be, will be. On the other hand, maybe you program for local training needs first, and only later develop formal credit courses. As long as your program is relevant, what difference should its form or range make?

Part of the problem for undergraduate gerontology arises from the graduate- or professional-level perspective of most of the existing literature relating to the issue of academic gerontology. In that perspective, the primary functions of academic gerontology seem not at all unclear: By a universal and practically absolute rationale, graduate centers and postgraduate institutes of gerontology know exactly what they are about. Witness the common functions of multidisciplinary centers anticipated in the Title IV-C guidelines. Compare the programs in gerontology found in the leading university centers in the

United States. To be sure, there are differences among university centers of gerontology. But, we also find in these centers a hard-core commonality of central, program-defining functions. These functions provide a stable context for interpreting quite logically and easily whatever is antecedent, ancillary, or even alternative to them as relative and devoid of universal and absolute structure. Thus, for example, undergraduate academic gerontology is free to do whatever it wants to do because ultimately whatever it does could never be considered a substitute for mainline graduate-level gerontology.

Part of the problem for undergraduate gerontology may also arise from the priorities of professional organizations like AGHE and the Gerontological Society. For example, AGHE, in favor of other concerns, has not yet structured for its membership a forum in which the analysis of academic gerontology on all levels could be pursued with direction and continuity. A standing committee on educational policy might provide such a forum. Similarly, the Committee on Education within the Gerontological Society has not yet organized a symposium or series of symposia on issues in undergraduate academic gerontology.

So much for the problem. Now, I want to comtemplate a solution. That brings me to the third aspect of the "Functions of Academic Gerontology," namely, insights from the past. In its original conception, gerontology was predominantly oriented to the production of the graduate-level interdisciplinary (Koller, 1962) social gerontologist and the post-graduate disciplinary specialist on aging. Toward that end, the best available students were sought for gerontological studies. Almost without exception, the original 76 trainees in the field aimed at an application of their newly acquired gerontological knowledge and skills on the graduate level of teaching, research, and administration (Donahue, 1960). In that pioneering context, the role of undergraduate academic gerontology was conceived as introductory and motivational vis-à-vis graduate studies. In the first instance, undergraduate studies on aging were to represent a loosely organized and broad background in the social, biological, and psychological aspects of aging. Subsequent graduate and post-graduate studies were to provide a generalized ("generalist") integration of those aspects and, ultimately (at the choice of the individual) a single-discipline specialization. Secondly, undergraduate courses in gerontology were to motivate students toward further graduate-level studies and career specialization.

The earliest reported undergraduate program of studies in gerontology did not adhere to that model (1962). It represented, instead, a fully developed undergraduate major which aimed at producing the "generalist" on aging closely akin to the social gerontologist of the graduate level. Symptomatically, that program also shied away from strict gerontology nomenclature and offered instead a major in sociology with a concentration in social gerontology. Other undergraduate programs have subsequently followed suit, with variations on that same theme. This approach has served to cloud rather than clarify the function(s) of academic gerontology on all levels of academe. Unwittingly, it has contributed to an attenuation of that quality of preservice gerontological preparation and expertise which from the beginning has been the goal of mainstream gerontological advocates. The issue, then, is whether the academic gerontological community endorses baccalaureate-level practice in the field of aging. Both the original insight of that community and the credentialing/licensure dynamic that is rapidly evolving (and is perhaps overdue) in many areas of gerontological practice seem to discourage such an endorsement. On the contrary, both that insight and that dynamic urge the defining and structuring of undergraduate gerontology almost exclusively as a propaedeutic to graduate-level training and credentialing. Does this mean there should be no terminal function for undergraduate academic gerontology? Yes, and no. There should be no terminal function in terms of an endorsed or advocated baccalaureate-level service entry and/or practice. On the other hand, there should very definitely be an endorsed and advocated terminal function in terms of liberal education.

Undergraduate academic gerontology should be primarily organized and supported for inculcating age awareness, life enhancement, and critical social participation. Primarily, it should aim at coproducing, with all other undergraduate disciplines, the humanized citizenry of the future, that body-politic of the late twentieth and early twenty-first century United States which will determine the context, criteria, and rewards of successful aging in the decades ahead. This rationale would motivate the programming and promotion of undergraduate gerontology predominately in terms of a broad range of gerontologized disciplinary and interdisciplinary elective courses, courses that relate to and organically accompany every major program of studies. As a foundation and/or complement to those courses, a basic course encompassing information about aging processes, social gerontology, and public policy on aging would be recommended. (Three separate core courses on those aspects should be available and/or required of those aspiring to graduate-level specialization and an eventual professional career in the field of aging.)

This proposed approach has a number of key advantages. First, it spares undergraduate gerontology the misplacement of energies and resources in the aping of a graduate and/or professional program of studies and training. Second, it integrates undergraduate gerontology into the liberalizing objectives of the undergraduate educational tradition. This latter has two major facets. On the one hand, it gives direction and impetus to the development of an interdisciplinary gerontological faculty from among existing faculty members (as distinct from the development/addition of a separate gerontology faculty). On the other hand, it opens the door to innovative, interdepartmental/interdivisional projects, including funding from sources other than the standard education training programs of the Administration on Aging. Finally, this approach serves to keep latter-day academic gerontology particularly faithful to the insights of its original seers and architects.

It seems to me that the college or university which structures undergraduate gerontology according to the rationale suggested here, and which supplements its program with elective interdepartmental films, conferences and colloquia, field trips, laboratory and/or experiential projects, will not only be doing something singularly innovative in academic gerontological circles, but will be demonstrating the organic, compatible link between academic gerontology's past and future. Such a college or university will be contributing to the life-span liberalizing/humanizing of future Americans by prioritizing a gerontological function that is specific to undergraduate education and for which there is no known substitute.

References

Bolton, C. R. Humanistic instructional strategies and retirement education programming. *Gerontologist*, 1976, *16*(6), 550–555.

College program in gerontology, announcement of, Mt. Angel College. *Geriatrics*, 1962, *17*(7), 100A.

Donahue, W. Training in social gerontology. *Geriatrics*, 1960, *15*(11), 801–809.

Freeman, J. T. Humanism and the humanities of aging. *Gerontologist*, 1976, *16*(2), 183–185.

Koller, M. Recommended curricula in social gerontology. *Geriatrics*, 1962, *17*(1), 260–264.

Seltzer, M. M. Education in gerontology: An evolutionary analogy. *Gerontologist*, 1974, *14*(4), 308–311.

Spinetta, J. J., and Hickey, T. Aging and higher education: The institutional response. *Gerontologist*, 1975, *15*(5), 431–435.

Tibbitts, C. Social gerontology. *Geriatrics*, 1960, *15*(10), 705–716.

Weg, R. B. Educational intervention and gerontology: An integration. *Gerontologist*, 1975, *15*(3), 448–451.

The Functions of Academic Gerontology

Mildred M. Seltzer
Miami University

The title of this particular discussion leaves us with words to define—*function* and *gerontologist*. The Random House dictionary defines *function* as an action or activity appropriate for a person, thing, or institution. The term also refers to public ceremonies. Further, a function is a factor related to or dependent upon other factors (1967). A final synonym for function is purpose.

It is less easy to find an adequate definition of *gerontology*. This same dictionary refers to it as the science dealing with aging and the special problems of aging persons. For our purposes, I consider gerontology a multidisciplinary endeavor which brings to bear the knowledge of a variety of sciences on a stage of life—namely, middle and old age but particularly old age. It differs from a single disciplinary view of an entire world, one which sees reality as atoms, social groups, or some other units of analysis.

I question whether academics in other disciplines question and discuss their functions to the same extent as do academic gerontologists. Wherefore is this field different from other fields? Are we implicitly expressing a social ideology when we raise the issue of whether we have functions and what these are? One questions whether any academic discipline has functions beyond those of developing, creating and transmitting knowledge. Is there a mission aspect to gerontology that is unique to the field or is this a question that applies to all academic disciplines (and, more fundamentally, are we a discipline)? Are the functions of academic gerontology different from those of academic chemistry, psychology, biology, physics, sociology? Moreover, do these functions of academic (whatever *academic* refers to) gerontology differ for the teaching and/or research faculty, academic administrators, or for practitioners? The answer to this question is probably yes. Academic gerontology is essentially the nonpractice, nonapplied aspect of the study of aging. Its data have been useful to but not necessarily created by the practitioner.

If we accept the foregoing, it is appropriate to assume that the functions of academic gerontology are different from the functions of the academic gerontologist. If academic gerontology can have any function at all, it has as its chief purpose the scientific study of aging. This study is carried on through research, in laboratories, and/or in any other appropriate way of sciencing. The functions of the academic gerontologist are to do research, to educate people, and to train them. Many academic gerontologists also define themselves as having the further functions of public service and advocacy.

From a research point of view, it is important to learn something about the nature of aging, to have some interplay between research, theory, and practice, and to eliminate the arbitrary distinction between pure and applied research.

From an educational point of view, there are a number of functions to be served in the academic environment. I have referred to several of these elsewhere. A major function is to communicate knowledge about the nature of aging (insofar as we know it) to students and others because aging is a normal part of the life cycle. If we teach something about early childhood and adulthood, then certainly it is consistent to teach about other periods and transitions in the life cycle. Such information can enable people to deal with their own eventual aging as well as the aging of family members and the aging of populations. It will also familiarize students with material which may be of value to them in their eventual professions and occupations. This is true whether the student is a doctor, lawyer, or merchant chief.

Courses in gerontology have another major implicit function. It is to demonstrate that academic disciplines have no real boundaries. There may be a beginning to knowledge but there certainly is no end to it. We may be able to divide college campuses into neat little buildings and separate little departments, each of which may be autonomous in a Balkanized version of a university. If we want to understand something about the nature of aging, however, we need the perspectives of many disciplines, not just that of one. Academic gerontology can to this extent serve as a model for multidisciplinary and interdisciplinary activities in colleges and universities. The breakdown of disciplinary walls is slow in coming and I doubt very much if gerontologists, like Joshua, will bring them tumbling, but we may be able to bring about an occasional crack.

The public service mission of colleges and universities is either implicitly or explicitly expressed in each individual school's mission statement. Academic gerontologists, in carrying out the mission of their colleges and universities, therefore, have a responsibility to provide such services. This can be accomplished by transmitting accurate information about the nature of aging. This can be communicated by direct transmission in nonclassroom situations, by serving on boards, by giving advice, particularly when it is requested, to organizations providing services for older Americans. Faculty can also assist in reviewing legislation and policy statements. As individuals they can decide whether or not to participate in writing political platforms, and indirectly implementing programs.

Gerontologists have for some time distinguished between education and training. The academic gerontologist can provide short-term training for practitioners—both paraprofessionals and professionals—for colleagues, and for the lay public. Here my assumption is that it is better for accurate information to be transmitted by people whose ethics demand accuracy and objectivity than by those whose ideology colors the data.

Almost inevitably in papers like this there is some discussion about whether universities and colleges have specific social welfare and service functions. Should courses for older people be offered by schools? Should old people be involved in determining the nature of gerontology programs or, at least, serving on the boards and giving advice for such activities? Let me take up each of these questions. Whether the university has a social service function is obviously a question to be answered by the particular school involved. I personally have grave questions about whether one can simultaneously be both social worker and academician, both therapist and teacher. These, however, are personal opinions which, while I am glad to share and support with some evidence, are not necessarily shared by others. The provision of educational opportunities for older people is not only mandatory by law in many states, but is consistent with the philosophy which says that there is a beginning but no end to learning.

Whether or not old people should, as members of the category "old people," be on advisory governing boards, research committees, or otherwise having policy-determining positions merely by virtue of being old is another question altogether. It is not clear that by virtue of being a member of a specific social category one is necessarily qualified to determine programs appropriate for that category. It is intriguing that we have a society in which the expert is valued because of his/her background and expertise, and at the same time we turn around and assume the nonexpert is automatically an expert by virtue of the fact that he/she has taken a certain drug, is old, has cancer, has been psychotic. The unique experience becomes the qualifying criterion for expertise and the experience automatically substitutes for knowledge. There is a line between educated expertise and experienced membership in a special category as a qualifying characteristic.

There are some who suggest that academic gerontologists have an advocacy role on behalf of older people. Once again, this is often a matter for decision on the part of the college, university, and/or the individual. Certainly, the advocacy role ill becomes some academic gerontologists while, on the other hand, it fits like a cloak around others.

The issues we are facing now with reference to both the functions of academic gerontology and education in gerontology have been coming to a head in recent years. We are at a watershed point when we must examine carefully and critically the long-range consequences of current decisions. In general those of us in academe tend to behave on a day-by-day basis, academic year-by-year, grant period-to-grant period, biennium-to-biennium basis. The choices we make in determining the functions of academic gerontology, not only at our own schools, but in general, set off a Markov chain. Current decisions are structuring our futures and limiting our alternatives. We are living the development of a profession and might benefit by drawing more from the sociology of professions. We need to understand something about the emergence of new professions, the up and coming issues of licensing and credentialing, the role of our multidisciplinary endeavors in disciplinary-based universities. We are in an expanding field and what is otherwise the contracting economic and social system of the university. Throughout its history, our society has been based on values and guided by principles related to an expanded system. All of us have been reared and socialized with the belief that there is no limit to our resources and potential. Now we are faced with the fact that our potential may be boundless but our resources are not.

I have started with the topic of what is an academic gerontologist. I am ending with more questions than I have answered. The functions which I have described above are current functions. What I am concerned with now are the future functions and directions of academic gerontology and academic geron-tologists. What are we creating in our performances? In view of what we are doing, is it proper to ask how a gerontologist differs from other -ologists? Have we and are we creating a new profession and new professionals? What is its nature, if this is what we are doing? Are we saying that in the beginning there was aging and now there is the gerontologist? One is tempted to say God must have loved the old as he made so many of them. Since he made so many of them, are we now developing a profession and its academic background in response to our perceptions of older people's needs? I don't know the answers to these questions, and in many instances I am not even sure what questions to ask. On the other hand, I once learned that while it is not incumbent upon one to complete a task, neither should one desist from undertaking it.

The Effect of the Extension of Life on Undergraduate Academic Gerontology

Jerome Kaplan
Ohio State University

Introduction

The extension of life into the oldest of years relates, among other factors, to:

1. Fulfillment of the biblical three score and 10 years which is close to the average accomplishment in the United States

2. Recognition of behavioral and sociological variables for attaining age 70 and older and their interplay with biological and genetic variables (Lawton and Gottesman, 1974; Goldfarb, 1967)

3. Attainment of the assumed 120-year age as the theoretical limit of man's length of life. Despite claims of extreme longevity in several other societies, U. S. scientists note the lack of sufficient scientific data to support these claims. One must look to individual societal reasons for such reporting (Medvedev, 1974)

4. Pursuing the extension of the 120-year life span potential (Hayflick, 1974)

5. Efforts to maximize one's capacity to be more independent than dependent in old years, and thereby decrease and/or eliminate the decrements of senescence which heretofore have been viewed as normal aging. Chronic brain syndrome (reported by some under the umbrage of senility) has been viewed as abnormal aging. The effects of either however may produce similarity in behavior and result in dependence on others (Goldfarb, 1967;

INFORMAL COMMENTARIES AND EXPLORATIONS

Barnes, Sack, and Shore, 1973; Kahn, 1975; Kahana and Coe, 1975; Redick, 1974; and Simon and Epstein, 1970).

Each of these items has a profound effect on permitted and possible life styles for those now living in the oldest of the years as well as those who will live. As a consequence of increased longevity, societal resources will be restructured. Existing programs will be refined and modified. Newer services will be developed. Retirement ages will be altered. Leisure will be rethought. Medical practice will have different values relating to the efficacy of procedures. Our acceptance of the old years will be different from what it has been at any time since the modern era in the United States.

Past

As we look at the history of gerontology we learn that prior to the 1600s the phenomena of old age were explained by magic, myth, and speculation. In 1000 B.C. the average age of life was 18 years. For hundreds of years thereafter it hovered around 25 years and consequently old age was an unusual occurrence subject to explanation only by people's imagination.

Gerontology, as the science of aging, began when people started inquiring about the characteristics of those who lived into the old years. Scientific inquiry was preceded by the antediluvian view. This approach was based on the belief that people lived to extreme old age in the time of the Old Testament. Subsequently the Greeks developed the hyperborean view which suggested the existence of a distant place where people lived to be very old. The rejuvenation view claimed that magical essences and/or techniques existed, if one could find them, which would rejuvenate people. These ideas continue to linger with us. Efforts still are undertaken by those who believe they can prove these notions.

The first efforts toward a scientific study of aging began with Francis Bacon who searched for a single cause of aging and Sir Francis Galton in the latter part of the nineteenth century. Prior to the nineteenth century, however, the study of aging was generally relegated to theological rather than scientific consideration and the number of inquiries into its nature were sparse.

There was an increased number of empirical approaches to aging early in the twentieth century. Investigation into the cause of longevity was introduced. There was an examination into concepts of psychological and behavior intervention as well as into the involvement of the central nervous system in aging. At this time, too, the distinction between normal and pathological old age was first introduced. This issue has still not been resolved. The earlier view that aging has one cause has increasingly given way to the view there are multiple determinants of aging: biological, behavioral, psychological, and sociological, each with independent components and each interdependent upon the other.

Present Status

Biochemists with theories having various degrees of potential are exploring the dream of postponing death and retarding aging. Our recognition of the social and political consequence of great numbers of people living into the old years is, however, in an embryonic stage. The psychological and behavioral implications and the concomitant unrefined social and political ones regarding a sizeable extension of life are touched upon by a number of independent investigators. A cohesive and integrated approach of the unknown individual and societal consequences, given a major breakthrough in longevity, has not yet taken place. To a large extent the lack of such an approach is due to the fact that researchers, practitioners, and policy makers each operate in separate milieus. Most of our modern social and psychological knowledge has not yet sifted to the citizenry due to its newness and the lack of an overall effort to transmit the information. Much knowledge has not been utilized by practitioners playing service roles because of the still unresolved issue of whether or not gerontology is to be a field unto itself or is to provide a body of knowledge for incorporation into other fields. As a result, properly educated and trained personnel have heretofore been few in number.

Biological scientists have problems in learning more about the causes and retardants of aging because of the lack of sufficient fundamental data. Additionally, research is complicated by the fact that biological changes with time affect almost all biological systems from the molecular level to the whole organism and it is therefore difficult to isolate the significant variables. Because of our on-and-off support of research about human aging, such research is not yet very sophisticated. The intermittent nature of this support has also resulted in limiting the number of researchers and extended research.

Although longitudinal studies with humans give us critical data of a different nature than do cross-sectional ones, the former studies have been few in number. The paucity of such studies is due to the U.S. cultural desire for immediate answers, which further relates to subsequent funding sources. In turn, court decisions have manifested culturally influenced agism. This is manifested by courts considering old age as a period of incompetency rather than by their acceptance of individualized capabilities of people who happen to be advanced in years.

Potential Future Developments

It is possible that within the next 15 years, biological research may result in the development of a unifying causal theory about aging. It seems probable that such a theory will be based upon the idea that genetic instability is a cause of aging and that the genetic contribution is the foremost factor in determining life span. During this same period of time, medical technology may advance in such a way as to allow for quick measurement of the rate of aging. This would result in the likelihood that people could fulfill their life spans. Equally important areas for research investigation are those relating to the evolvement of an ethic for extending life at one end of the life cycle while simultaneously decreasing the number of births at the other end. It would also be essential to examine the extent of qualitative essence to life in the old years in order that our society's old people contribute to society rather than be dependent upon it (Bok, 1974).

The continued, gradual increase in the average life expectancy, much less the attainment of the limits of life span, will produce 70- and 80-year-olds with the energy of those currently in their 50's and 60's. It will also produce greater numbers of people subject to the infirmities of the aging process in their 90's, 100's, and 110's as well as to pathological aging. These changes will both magnify the ambiguities and uncertainties in the roles of the elderly and will, simultaneously, provide greater numbers of both dependent and independent people.

Those who will continue to be independent and to find new ways of contributing to society will do so through the triad of household, voluntary service, or part-time work. It will require intensive educational orientation both formal and informal at all levels of schooling to change cultural views about old age held by the old as well as the others. It will necessitate the introduction of content about aging into our elementary schools through the higher educational system which trains teachers. *It further suggests direct aging courses and aging content be a requisite in every undergraduate sequence.*

Because of the susceptibility of aging per se as well as pathological aging, a greater number of people will be mentally impaired 15 years hence than ever before as the average age of life creeps up. To combat this great dependency inherent in the extension of life, intensive research, demonstration, and service support should be undertaken to learn and to treat the causes of confusion and senility. In this context, biological and medical research will then focus more finitely on a bio-causation while psychosocial research would be freer to pinpoint causations and remedies in its arena. Current trends suggest that the proponents of both orientations will within 15–20 years find that there is multiple causation of these symptoms. We need to develop, within the next 20 years, easy-to-use, valid diagnostic tools which will enable us to intervene and prevent symptoms of senility and confusion. The development of such tools will have a a direct bearing on changing our society's negative views of older people as being dependent. The new cultural definition instead, will be one of the aged as independent functioning people.

Despite demonstration of what can be done to contain mental impairments affecting independent functioning, it has been a gerontological and geriatric plague that these demonstrations have no continuity of support. There is, for example, a psychogenic concept of a senility spiral which sees the loss of role as a major first step, with each subsequent step leading toward a lessened feeling of self-worth and the eventual end in death (Barnes et al., 1973). The extent to which bio-gerontologists as compared with psycho/social gerontologists would accept this view is, perhaps, self-evident.

A high percentage of confused older people now reside permanently in nursing homes. In some instances, the nursing home environment causes rather than cures the confusion. This occurs despite our knowledge about how environmental stress affects behavior (Kaplan, 1974).

While many would argue that if no one had sufficient funds in the old years, all else could be handled, the view is presented here that in the long run full acceptance of an old person is even more critical and important than sufficient funds. While some believe confusion is bio-based and others that it is social in origin, the view expressed here is that it may be caused by either or by both in varying degrees of concert.

Discussion

It is possible to establish an extensive catalogue of moral and immoral actions with respect to the treatment of the aged. Such actions as the following illustrate this (Kaplan, 1974):

1. *Negotiation or imposition of treatment options;*
2. *Provision of adequate or inadequate nutrition;*
3. *Maintenance or disregard of patient privacy;*
4. *Promotion or restriction of unnecessary institutionalization;*
5. *Therapeutizing or dehumanizing treatment methodologies;*
6. *Processing or neglect of patient care, including the inability of a physician to visit a nursing home patient;*
7. *Servicing or exploitation of patient deficits;*
8. *Provision or disregard of safety and security measures;*
9. *Professionalizing or desensitizing treatment personnel;*
10. *Unifying or compartmentalizing related treatment resources;*
11. *Liberation or prolongation of patient dependencies; and*
12. *Provision or withholding of related treatment supports or resources.*

Lawmakers, who through funding of service provision make it possible or difficult to act within this ethical construct, have defined old age through social security. Consequently, many people have become old as they conform to the attitudes and expectations of the legal decision that 65 is old.

The social implications of aging are inherently related to societal values. Changes in values will result from an amassment of knowledge, its transmission and its utilization. The key change in views will occur when that segment of the elderly, who are the great dependents in both cost and imagery, can retain or regain their independence and mental competence. The expectations attributed to the legal age of 65 then can be overthrown.

Recommendations

Toward this end, the single most important attribute of life's extension in the next decades is to change the image of old age. One key to this is the removal of the senility symbolism. Another is knowledge transmission. It is, then, suggested that:

1. All undergraduate education require a core of specific aging content courses, to include basic biological, behavioral, psychological, and sociological gerontology.

2. All undergraduate professional degree offerings be required to offer a gerontological concentration as one of its options.

3. Gerontological technician training be the purview of the technical colleges and institutes and gerontological knowledge transmission be the responsibility of the colleges and universities.

4. The models of other professions be critically analyzed to insure gerontological input. There need not be disparity between the view of "we need gerontologists" and "we need professionals with gerontological expertise." Neither is there disparity in the views that one can be a B.A. gerontologist and a graduate gerontologist. We have, for example, R.N.'s and social workers with differing responsibilities.

Knowledge transmission in the psychosocial realm will remove a basic barrier in attaining ontological stature for old age, making it equal to all others. It will underpin an ethical construct for acceptance of human uniqueness in the oldest of years and allow for the overthrow of the self-fulfilling prophecy of legal old age.

If there will be millions in their 90's in the foreseeable future, then there must be more old people as contributors rather than noncontributors and liabilities to society. Only this can keep the old from being in open confrontation with the young for society's available resources. Academic undergraduate gerontology will play a prime role in achieving this solution.

References

Barnes, E. K., Sack, A., and Shore, H. Guidelines to treatment approaches: Modalities and methods for use with the aged. *Gerontologist*, 1973, *14*(1), 37–45.

Bok, S. Commentary. In L. R. Tancredi (Ed.), *Ethics of health care*. Washington, D.C.: National Academy of Science, 1974, 304–313.

Goldfarb, A. T. Geriatric psychiatry. In A. Freedman and H. I. Kaplan (Eds.), *Comprehensive textbook of psychiatry*. Baltimore: Williams and Wilkins Co., 1967, 1564–1587.

Hayflick, L. The strategy of senescence. *Gerontologist*, 1974, *14*(1), 37–45.

Kahana, E., and Coe, R. M. Alternatives in long-term care. In Sylvia Sherwood (Ed.), *Long-term care: A handbook for researchers, planners and providers*. New York: Halsted Press Division of John Wiley & Sons, 1975, 511–572.

Kahn, R. L. The mental health system and the future aged. *Gerontologist*, 1975, *15*(1), 24–31.

Kaplan, J. In search of policies for care of the aged. In L. R. Tancredi (Ed.), *Ethics of health care*. Washington, D.C.: National Academy of Science, 1974, 281–308.

Lawton, M. P., and Gottesman, L. E. Psychological services to the elderly. *American Psychologist*, 1974, *29*(1), 689–693.

Medvedev, Z. A. Caucasus and altay longevity: A biological or social problem? *Gerontologist*, 1974, *14*(5), 381–387.

Redick, R. S. Patterns in use of nursing homes by the aged mentally ill. *Statistical Note 107*. Rockville, Md.: Biometry Branch NIMH, 1974.

Simon, A., and Epstein, L. J. Alternatives to mental hospital care for the geriatric patient. *Current Psychiatric Therapies*, 1970, *10*, 225–231.

Developing and Emerging Programs in Gerontology: First Steps in Program Development

Ruth B. Weg
University of Southern California

There has been considerable discussion about direction in education for gerontology, about the necessity for excellence, about the particular form and content for the hard and soft dollar and competition related thereto. There have been admonitions to regard the research bases of disciplines more seriously. Concern for how many programs, how much is enough, has raised the suggestion that growth in gerontology may be reaching some asymptote—some plateau.

May I respectfully note relating to the never-ending search for the dollars necessary to mount, maintain, and move forward, that those who were committed to the field years ago have made the current market place. We can and must continue to actively participate in shaping the market place.

There is no alternative to "fired up" imagination, to the willingness to take a chance, to the more than lip service to heterogeneity, creativity, and diversity that will protect this multidiscipline against the stagnation and obsolescence of respectability, predictability, and security.

By all means—let the development of programs proceed with care, with justification, with clarity and evaluation. Let history be a teacher, but go frequently to the "crystal ball." No market analysis of products bought from the grocery shelf has ever been useful in indicating "what hitherto unseen packaging" will take off.

How Much Is Enough

Some have suggested that there may now be more than enough programs for gerontology in institutions of higher learning. My own guess is that gerontology may have just come of age. It is too soon to put a cap on the growth of centers. There may indeed be some merit in "bigger is not necessarily better." However, systematic investigations of program strengths, emphases, evaluations, excellence, and gaps have not been undertaken. Much more dialogue and data are required before all who would drink from the well are sent packing.

Rigors of Research, Excellence

In answer to the call for return to the rigors of our disciplines—may I suggest "we never left home." There is no disagreement. There must be a continuing flow of knowledge which remains the basis for teaching, for decision making, for the development of practice. There may be only the caution, that in our objective research, we occasionally lift our eyes to the *persons* involved in the process.

And finally to the call for excellence—for criteria—for evaluation, amen. However, may I remind us, that as with love and motherhood, there may be no singular route to the virtues of excellence and appropriateness in gerontology.

The questioning, the ongoing search that characterizes all who have gathered in the educational community are not only stimulating—but a lifeline to the health of gerontology. Differences of opinion and the consequent ferment is the medium that permits the next step in growth from all the available input at any one point in time. Only in the sterility of stasis and at last in death, is the energy and turning at an end. Consensus could drain this energy early in development.

Program Development: Ambience and Activities

The climate for development in which we find ourselves—from educational and gerontological perspectives—has been explored. We are all aware of the ambiguity of the realities presented, and our ambivalent reactions.

However, there is little doubt among any of us that gerontology has created a niche in institutions of higher learning. As recently as 10 years ago, perhaps eight programs in gerontology could have been considered active centers of research, education, and community programs in gerontology. You have heard, according to the *National Directory of Educational Programs in Gerontology*, there are 1,275 entries of educational programs, as of July 1976, with a focus in aging, all in various stages and states of development. Although a number of these programs are still working hard to stay in the same place, you have heard repeated recitation of those who have grown and prospered, in the student populations served, faculty involved, and in visible achievements.

Ten years ago, the educational emphases in aging were largely in university centers and programs committed primarily to research and doctoral training. Today, there are additional concentrations of effort in community programs and in multilevel educational programs across the country. Programs exist for the baccalaureate, masters, certificate, professional, para-professional, and for the older person. Doctoral and postdoctoral programs continue, with degrees coming from the discipline, the dissertation in gerontology, as part of the effort that must go on to enlarge our data base and specialization in aging.

There is no single shape and scope of gerontological education that is "the model" from which all others must be molded. Each development is unique. There is generally a "fit" with the particular strengths, interests, and availability of faculty, needs of students, and the community. Other aspects are the moral and financial support of institutional administration as well as potential and actual monies from a variety of private and public sources. It is inescapable that large numbers of institutions of higher learning have finally accepted gerontology as a legitimate academic concentration, as an area of scholarship, inquiry, and practice.

Additional significant evidence of the growth of gerontology is in the accumulation of real knowledge—disciplinary and interdisciplinary, related to the processes and mechanisms of aging which can be applied in theory and practice. This knowledge is organized in a variety of forms—not only with multiplication of monographs, journals, and series, but in films, tapes, conference proceedings, etc.

There have been some major trends that must be considered as supportive of continued growth in gerontology. Researchers and educators and other professionals committed to aging no longer see gerontology as an auxiliary source of activity and monies, but as a major work in their careers. The continual improvement toward excellence in all their efforts attests to the pride and pleasure associated with primary identity on the part of scientists and practitioners.

There is the dramatic increase in the number of older adults in this country. Never before have there been so many older persons who belie the myths and stereotypes of the invalid, medical model. In reality, they are healthier, better educated, and more demanding than earlier generations of oldsters—and many are organized, vocal, and effective advocates; e.g., AARP/NRTA, NCOA, Gray Panthers, National Institute of Senior Centers, International Senior Centers, International Senior Citizens.

The activities of government agencies have also picked up momentum: In a trajectory begun with the Older Americans' Act of 1965, and assorted amendments, there exists a wide range of programs for and with older persons, educational programs in gerontology and a network of state and area agencies on aging. The unbelievable spread of such activities can be seen in part in the 620 designated planning and service areas throughout the United States.

In belated response to the 1961 and 1971 White House Conferences on Aging commitments and promises—programs for and with older persons have proliferated. The Administration on Aging has served as a major conduit of governmental support to the state and area agencies related to aging, and also to the educational efforts at institutions of higher learning. At times, the conduit has been a slow moving, erratic flow of information and monies, clogged, no doubt, by the quixotic state of the Office of Management and Budget and the unstable, federal administration as a whole in the recent past.

Another source of governmental support for so-called hard science research and research training was the National Institute for Child Health and Human Development with only 10 percent of the budget of that agency earmarked for the study of aging. Finally, in May of 1976, Robert Butler, sensitive, experienced, and committed to gerontology and the needs of older persons, became head of the National Institute on Aging—an agency that was another belated response to the 1971 White House Conference on Aging. There is good reason to feel that in Dr. Butler aging has an active advocate for gerontology in research, education, and translation of knowledge into practice for and with older persons.

In 1974 the Veterans Administration created Regional Geriatric Research Educational and Clinical Center Programs to develop, demonstrate, and institute quality care programs specific to VA community systems, providing extended care to elderly citizens.

The media have been stirring from their slumber, too. Radio, TV, films, magazines, and newspapers—in straight news or editorial programming, in interviews and stories—are involved in gerontology. They are talking about age and sexuality, memory and aging, the middle-aged and older woman, later-life love relationships and marriage, and television is obviously employing more older persons in presentations. None of this could have happened even five years ago.

Educational pace setting goes on in the environment of confused and confusing federal and state support to aging programs. This is supported by the ever-increasing visibility and confidence among groups of older persons. The end result is impact upon the media and institutional world around us. Gerontology, even in its struggle for visibility and competence, has contributed to the change that is emerging. We did not wait for the "market analysis," but became part of the developing picture.

Ambivalence remains in educational communities about disciplinary or multidisciplinary designs, about centers, institutes, or programs, and at what levels. Nevertheless, there is a definite shift from the tentative, insecure position of the earlier days, only five to eight years ago, to an identification with the expanding, pioneering area that is gerontology.

Our concerns have moved from acceptance to more productive issues. These include: curricula, basic and applied research, personnel needs, collegial relationships, and student interests and needs. With an eye to the future we must consider the following: potential employment of those in educational programs, real needs and wants of the community of currently older persons and those who will be old in the near future, communication, transmission, and publication of information for the different consuming publics and with the particular requirements and monies of the educational institution.

This would appear to be a very good time to emphasize the techniques that will change the attitudes and mores of the society related to aging. We must see to it that information about *normal aging* and the *continued growth of human capacities throughout life* are integrated into the moral and mental fibre of everyone in this country. A more accurate notion of the life continuum serves the young, the middle aged, and the old as it slowly moves the decision makers into a more realistic, responsible stance with a significant portion of the electorate.

This is a good time to develop a life cycle perspective to legitimate the middle and later years of life. Such a perspective would assign to the study of later life stages the intellectual energy and monies correctly accorded to earlier stages of life—infancy, childhood, adolescence, and youth. This is a good time to turn theory into practice, and wash out the mythology of aging as only invalidism, loneliness, inadequacy, and brain deterioration.

Unlike most disciplines and college departments, gerontology represents a field of positive growth—in educational, institutional commitments, in practice orientation, in the accumulation of data and theoretical concepts, and in the search for answers to basic questions.

This is a time of significant growth in professional organizations for gerontology. The American Gerontological Society now has over 4,200 members, roughly double that of eight years ago. There are now 12 state societies and two major regional conferences. And there is, of course, this relatively new organization for institutional membership, the Association for Gerontology in Higher Education. Its development is a direct function of the growth of programs in institutions of higher learning. There is also the acceleration of gerontological activity in other parts of the world, in international organizations for gerontology and geriatrics.

The Steps for Developing and Emerging Programs

Developing and emerging programs in gerontology and their faculties have many options for direction and contribution—into nearly virgin territory, or into greater depth on issues and structure of human development and aging. In every case, there will be particular steps to legitimation and growth. Among the large number of steps will be the following: acceptance by an educational community, efforts to be viewed as cooperative not competitive with traditional disciplines, the identification of more than moral support, the core of faculty, administrators, and students pulling together in the creation and acceptance of courses, the development of rewards comparable to those from the more usual academic areas, the ongoing examination of goals, specific objectives, criteria, and evaluative tools. The sequence is dependent on a set of circumstances. The talent, commitment, and interest of a critical number of faculty and potential students would appear to be minimum requirements for the developing program. Talent and commitment, however important as a nucleus for growth, are frustrated without the financial and moral support of institutional administration.

Resources increase daily: in educational materials of all kinds, at many levels, in scientific search for new information, in potential colleagues who have already completed substantial works and study in aging, in programs for and with older persons, and in the numbers of students of many ages ready to participate. A variety of governmental agencies at city, state, and federal levels are at work in the field of aging with informational and financial supports. Many untried agencies require socialization into the field and many private foundations as well. Admittedly, the currently available funds are not what is required to implement the programs that shall effect the hoped-for changes in the development of new knowledge, in the transmission of that knowledge, in the translation into practice, and finally into the lives of older persons—but there is tomorrow.

Developing and emerging programs have the opportunity and the responsibility to help define the present state of the arts and sciences that make up gerontology and contribute to its future. Gerontology as a multidiscipline has evolved through a variety of stages in its life cycle: an area of concentration, a specialization, an area for research, a degree, a major, an art, a practice, a multidiscipline.

When we meet again three or four years from now, the study, the education, and the community programs may have forged another stage. No program will walk the identical path of any other—nor is that desirable. Even a cursory examination of the phenomenal increase in programs in institutions of higher learning is testimony to the heterogeneity that is reasonable and fortunate. We have moved past the search for the monolithic "best" to the recognition that a pluralistic society and its people are best served with pluralism in patterns of knowledge gathering, transmission of new information, and translation into practice.

There will be difficulties and even failures, as well as exciting successes. The growing presence of representatives of countless programs at professional meetings within the last few years provides the most recent evidence for confidence in constructive growth, whatever unique blueprint is followed. We cannot predict a future—but we must anticipate. There are no guarantees, nor would they profit us. The future in gerontology is assured—the definitive frameworks remain to be detailed, hopefully with enough of the details yet to be written as we go. We are all responsible.

Little learning takes place from engagement with a finished product—education is at its potential best when the learners are involved with shaping and using the processes of inquiry. Gerontology began its days as an academic reality in the hands and minds of those who chose to take a chance into a relatively unformed, unproven area—like the turtle whose long life could be one of the symbols of gerontology. The educator and scientist James B. Conant has told us that even the turtle makes progress only when he sticks his neck out.

First Steps in Program Development: Developmental Tasks

Harvey L. Sterns
The University of Akron

A number of important vectors have come together to produce an increased interest in the field of aging and new demands on postsecondary education. First is the growth of the older segment of the population. Second is the increased interest in research in life-span development and gerontology. Third is the increased funding from federal, state, and local agencies for education and training in the field of aging. Fourth is the dramatic increase in agencies and institutions providing direct services to older people. These include federal agencies, state commissions on aging, area agencies on aging, local government offices, planning agencies, multipurpose senior centers, senior service agencies, preretirement preparation programs, senior housing units and planned retirement communities, long-term care facilities, nutrition sites, and numerous other paid and volunteer organizations.

With the increase in service agencies and programs, the need for workers and administrators with training in gerontology is present at the paraprofessional, administrative, technical, and professional levels. There is an immediate need to augment the training of in-service personnel and the inclusion of such training in the preservice preparation of our students in existing degree programs. There is as a result an increasing need for college-level researchers and teachers to carry out the training and education of potential and current workers in the field.

Over the last few years educational institutions have had increased opportunities to offer workshops and seminars, noncredit courses, credit courses for both preservice and in-service students. In a number of states, active training officers from state commissions on aging have helped to stimulate educational opportunities using state and local Title III and IV-A funds. Some educational institutions have found this to be an exciting challenge and natural extensions of ongoing programs, others have had to be dragged in, and other institutions have failed to become involved at all. The responses of particular educational institutions are, of course, determined by interest, history, and faculty strength. There are a number of mature programs in gerontology in this country, some going back to right after World War II. However, the vast majority of educational institutions find themselves presently responding to these new demands.

A small number of faculty who were trained in established programs find the development of gerontology education a natural expression of their training. Very often these faculty have been hired in traditional departmental settings and have begun to develop relevant course work, degree programs, and in some cases university-wide programs. Each individual and institution seem to have their own developmental history. Other faculty are now deciding to add the specialty of adulthood and aging to previous training. The impetus provided by expanded interest in gerontology can serve as an important stimulus for growth of individuals and programs not caught up in earlier opportunities.

Regardless of the particular history of faculty and institution, it is imperative to have educational and training programs of high quality. There is a great concern about the increasing number of "instant" gerontologists and resulting programs. It is imperative that in a field that must overcome so much misinformation and long held stereotypes that the latest information is presented. In a fast changing field with a constantly evolving research base, we must have well trained, actively involved faculty. Even current texts promote out-of-date views; thus, continued study, research, and professional involvement become key foci. One of the most exciting aspects of gerontology in various disciplines is the dynamic change in the knowledge base, and opportunities to contribute new research. There is a great danger in self-styled gerontologists promoting obsolete views. Even the most competent in primary disciplines should engage in special training to become involved at a professional level in gerontology. Fortunately, a number of professional societies and academic institutions have been offering continuing education and advanced training in gerontology for faculty and advanced students.

In our education and training we want to provide information about normal aging as experienced by the majority of our older adult population. At the same time we want to prepare individuals to deal with the increased number of older adults who have special physical, emotional, and/or economic wants and needs. The percentage of older adults experiencing normal aging and longer lives on the average will increase but the number of special populations will increase in absolute number and make increased demand on already overtaxed services.

The most basic question is "Does an individual faculty member, department, college, or university want to become involved in developing educational programs in the field of aging?"

If the answer is yes, some faculty involvement in gerontology may start with the opportunity to develop a new course or to develop new research involvements. This takes the form of a personal commitment. For others, there may be the opportunity to develop with colleagues an option in an existing training program or develop a totally new program. In this case departmental and university support must be solicited.

In other educational institutions the impetus may come from members of the board of trustees, the president of the university, deans, or department heads who feel that the institution should begin to develop a program. Whatever the stimulus, the tasks placed on faculty to develop such programs are very much the same.

Atchley and Seltzer (1977) in *Developing Educational Programs in the Field of Aging* raise the question: Where to start? They state, "There are some basic questions to be asked and answered: Is there adequately trained faculty? Is there faculty support for this undertaking? Is there administrative support? Are funds available to build up library facilities? Is there potential student interest? Is program being considered namely because there may be outside funds available?" (page 3).

If the answer to these basic questions points to further development, a number of additional questions and steps can be dealt with.

1. What is the nature and degree of training available in your geographic area? One should be clearly aware of what is available at other institutions to avoid unwanted duplication. It is possible in some areas that similar training at a number of institutions is warranted or the possibility of cooperative programs should also be explored when possible. A careful assessment of the needs and wants of in-service community practitioners is one starting place. Workshops and noncredit courses can serve as experimental ground for faculty developing their skills in this new area. This is not to imply that workshops and noncredit courses do not demand high level of knowledge and special training; however, these usually short-term situations allow for explorations into the best approaches of presenting new information. Careful evaluation can lead to immediate feedback which in turn can lead to improved teaching approaches. Experience gained at this level can be translated into sections of existing courses or cause new courses to be implemented at the undergraduate and graduate levels.

2. Who are the faculty at your institution willing to become involved in supporting an adulthood and aging program? A core of interested faculty may be easily targeted and this group can serve as a nucleus for a faculty committee. However, a wise step is to carry out a campus-wide survey of faculty interest. The number and diversity of interest of faculty is usually quite surprising and often talented and trained people are discovered in other

departments who were not previously known to the core group. When one has this information, it becomes possible to begin discussion regarding the development of new courses or parts of courses in the home departments of interested faculty. It is also possible to begin discussion about how these courses in home departments can be linked into a meaningful sequence of courses which can become the basis for a minor or certificate program.

Simultaneously, there can be careful study of already existing programs. Each school is unique in that often how one starts and the nature of the approach will be determined by talent available. Often it becomes apparent that a specially trained new faculty member may be needed. This realization is important because it may be able to be implemented when new faculty are hired or it may influence faculty members to undergo retraining. The use of consultants from established programs and interaction with other programs through national associations and regional groups may accelerate the process because of opportunities to utilize experience gained in other settings. This process of exploring and developing a program in gerontology will be most effective if cooperation and involvement of department heads, deans, and other university administration are present early in the developmental process. Faculty may be very pleasantly surprised at the cooperation they may receive. The formalization of a program in gerontology can take many forms at department, college, or all-college or university levels. Some universities have set up institutes or centers early in development with key faculty to coordinate and help develop the effort for the units involved. At other institutions the establishment of a center or institute comes about as a natural progression in the growth of the department, college, and total institutional involvement. This depends on the level of support that the institution is willing to provide for the project and/or the ability of the faculty involved to write grants which will provide funding for such development. The key element is faculty interest and administrative support. Whatever the level of development, the major concern should be with quality. Are able faculty involved? Are they involved in research related to gerontology? Are they involved in presenting their work in scholarly forums and in appropriate journals? Are faculty involved in community service and training related to gerontology? All of these areas can serve as indicators of professional development on the part of faculty.

3. What are the opportunities for your educational institution to interface with community groups? Cooperation with the area agency on aging, city, county, and state organizations may provide opportunities for support of training, research, and/or service. Community advisory groups can help colleges and universities to design workshops, noncredit and credit courses which will meet the needs of in-service personnel and at the same time provide new training opportunities for preservice students. Cooperation with senior centers, housing authorities, long-term care facilities, nutrition programs, and community service agencies may provide opportunities for mutu-

ally beneficial research and evaluation studies, joint service programs, and opportunities to place students in meaningful practicum and internship placements. Cooperation with local groups such as senior centers, special interest senior citizen groups, local chapters of American Association of Retired Persons and National Retired Teachers Association among others can lead to the development of educational opportunities for older adults. See Claeys (1976) for discussion of many of these issues.

4. What are the unique strengths that your education institution and faculty have to compete in regional, state, and federal research and training programs? A careful analysis of individual faculty interests as well as the ability to assemble multidisciplinary research teams can play an important role here. Faculty should arrange with their campus coordinators of research to be notified concerning research and training grants. Even better, key faculty should be placed on mailing lists of appropriate state and federal agencies such as Administration on Aging, National Institute on Aging, National Institute on Mental Health. See Cohen and Oppedisano-Reich (1977) for listing of government agencies and private foundations such as the Andrus Foundation of the American Association of Retired Persons and National Retired Teachers Association. Even if faculty are not ready to mount grants immediately, it helps to see what potential resources and areas are available. Be prepared for the short lead times by planning ahead projects of interest. Such funding is helpful only when it provides opportunities to grow in desired directions.

5. What are the opportunities to develop special programs and lectures for faculty, students, and community groups? An excellent way to increase the knowledge of faculty, students and community groups is to offer a lecture series in gerontology. If possible, nationally known experts can provide exciting first exposures for faculty and students. Also, their advice and counsel on program development as well as informal discussion with members of faculty and administration can greatly help to shape program development. Local talent both on and off campus should also be maximized through formal lectures and class presentations. Special projects such as preretirement education for faculty and staff, local industry, and general community may offer a real service and provide a meaningful sphere of involvement for interested faculty. The development of a lecture series for older adults about aging presented in the community can be a very worthwhile endeavor.

6. Are there ways that older adult groups and community agencies can help college and university development? The answer is definitely yes. It may be possible to utilize employees from the C.E.T.A. programs, Title IX program, or volunteers from groups such as the Retired Senior Volunteer Program. The help received from such programs may greatly help in dealing with manpower needs when institutional resources are limited. Also, it is possible that older adult groups may wish to help by offering financial support in the form of scholarship or gifts to the college or university.

These represent only a small number of possible questions, but they are among the more important for early stages of development. Keep in mind that as your program develops and grows and new components are added that the complexities increase accordingly. As things progress and support increases from the institution and from grants received, new developmental tasks become the order of the day. How do you maintain faculty involvement and interest on a long-term basis? How do you coordinate an ever increasing number of faculty and meet the needs of a growing number of students? How do you maintain quality instruction and programs? These are what I call good problems—problems or challenges that result from growth and development. I hope that you will have the opportunity to experience the challenge and excitement of some of these good problems.

References

Atchley, Robert C., and Seltzer, Mildred M. *Developing educational programs in the field of aging.* Oxford, Ohio: Scripps Foundation Gerontology Center, 1977.

Claeys, Russell R. *Utilization of college resources in gerontology: A program guide.* (Beverly Schwartz, Ed.). Upper Montclair, N.J.: Montclair State College, 1976.

Cohen, Lilly, and Oppedisano-Reich, Marie. *A national guide to government and foundation funding sources in the field of aging.* Garden City, N.Y.: Adelphi University Press, 1977.

Toward the Development of
Certification Programs in Gerontology

Lorin A. Baumhover
University of Alabama

The broad scope of this topic, "Sequence of Education/Training at the A.A., B.A., M.A., Ph.D. Levels," makes it extremely unlikely that a proper treatment of all these areas will be possible. As a result, I will limit my remarks to one model of providing graduate education, and more specifically, graduate training at the Specialist or Certificate level with special reference to new and emerging programs. I would like to discuss four areas: (1) one administrative model which is currently operating at the University of Alabama, (2) internal (academic) considerations in developing gerontology programs, (3) external (nonacademic) considerations, and (4) some general policy comments about developing gerontology programs.

1. Alabama Model

First, the Alabama experience. In 1971, the School of Social Work cosponsored the state grass roots hearings for the upcoming White House Conference on Aging. Later in the year, the School contracted with the Alabama Commission on Aging to conduct the Social Indicators Study of the aged for the state. As an outgrowth of these activities and later involvement with other state agencies, the Center for the Study of Aging was organized and began operations in 1972. The organizational model for the Center approximates a model earlier developed for other Centers within the University. The

School or department retains its administrative control over a Center, but program and policy input is provided through two University-wide committees, the Policy and Program Advisory Committees. This University-wide involvement has been particularly helpful to us in the aging center in the development of research and training proposals, in joint appointments, and in the development of gerontology courses in other departments. In addition, this model allows for clean lines of authority and helps to clarify rank, tenure, and promotion standards within a single administrative unit. More subtly, it provides some protection from the vicissitudes of soft funding.

Since 1972, the Center has received financial support from the Alabama Commission on Aging and from the University. More recently, however, support funds have been provided by the Administration on Aging through Title IV-A (Career Training) and through Title IV-C (Multidisciplinary Center of Gerontology) grants.

At the present time, the Center sponsors 10 research projects, directly funding five faculty research projects and five graduate student research projects. In addition, we have completed a number of other contracted research projects including evaluations of Title VII programs, needs assessments, and attitudinal studies. In the areas of education we are offering two undergraduate courses in gerontology and five on the graduate level which lead to the Specialist in Gerontology Certificate.

With this general description in mind, let us turn to some of the developmental or organizational components involved in setting up gerontology programs in higher education, particularly looking at ways where programs can be developed with a minimum of funds. First, some internal (academic) considerations.

2. Internal Considerations (Academic)

Early in the development of our Center we were faced with three major problems: (1) limited course offerings, (2) limited funds—soft funds, and (3) insufficient academic legitimacy.

1. Course Offerings. In 1971 only one undergraduate course in aging was offered within the University of Alabama. This was not a unique situation, certainly not unique to Alabama and I don't suspect unique to other universities in the nation. In addition to only one course offering, no other university or college within the state was offering more than one course, much less a degree program in the field of gerontology.

We were under contract at that time to provide training and technical assistance to developing Area Agencies on Aging and to other aging network personnel. After traveling the state on a workshop circuit, agency personnel began to request more formal training in gerontology. Certificates of attendance were "nice" to hang on the wall and Continuing Education Units

(CEU's) were of marginal usefulness as most individuals already held a bachelor's degree. As a result, agency personnel began requesting formal coursework in gerontology to be offered at off-campus locations at times and places where they could attend.

During this time we reviewed various program offerings, degree programs, training packages, and related courses that were currently available throughout the U.S. After this review we developed courses that responded both to program and academic needs such as one dealing with the implementation and evaluation of aging programs and another on the political and economic aspects of aging. These courses were guided through the appropriate university committees and approved. This was possible in large measure to agency pressure for more trained personnel in aging programs. These five courses have subsequently been revised, modified, and now constitute the courses required for the Specialist in Gerontology Certificate. They are: The Aging Process, Political-Economic Aspects of Aging, Research in Aging, Aging and Health Care, and Implementation and Evaluation of Programs for Older Adults.

2. *Limited Funds – Soft Funds.* The problem of limited funds remains a continuing concern to most centers, bureaus, institutes, and academic departments. Not being unique may make one feel better but it fails to have program benefits. I have never believed poverty has any uplifting moral qualities. I would like to share some ideas about developing programs even when faced with limited funds.

It is sometimes possible to generate joint appointments with existing academic departments without any transfer of funds. For example, we were able to develop joint [appointments] with the departments of Consumer Sciences, Sociology, and Human Development by simply asking the faculty members we desired and their respective deans if they would serve as joint appointments with the Center on Aging. At the present time three faculty members teach courses with gerontological content in their respective departments and have joint appointments with the Center.

In addition to joint appointments, additional program benefits may be realized by attempting to influence choices for new appointments in other departments on campus. Here, individuals with a secondary specialization or interest in gerontology may be suggested to fill an open position. This may be done indirectly by making other departments aware of research and funding opportunities in gerontology. One's ability to influence choice of appointments may vary widely and may meet with opposition, but by making your intentions known future choices may be influenced.

Another consideration is to develop cooperative relationships with your division of Continuing Education—extended programs section. In Alabama, the University's division of extended programs will pay for a regular on-campus course to be taught at an off-campus location if a sufficient number of students can be generated. The gerontology program can effectively be translated beyond the campus to areas where no education in gerontology is being offered at no cost to your program. Although not the national trend, some extended programs will recruit students, will provide registration materials, will help find a site, will collect the tuition, and will reimburse the course instructor. In some institutions it is even possible for regular courses to be offered on an on-campus basis, such as during weekends, interim terms, minimesters, nights, or compressed summer sessions and be paid for by Continuing Education.

In addition to regular courses, aging programs generate additional community support for their workshop activities and technical assistance projects. By taking advantage of their location in an institution of higher education, gerontology programs should automatically provide CEU's for workshops and training sessions. Although CEU's are not too useful in academic programs, some state agencies require a specified number of training contact hours to be completed every year, particularly in the health areas. Another way to increase your program thrust without additional revenue deals with increasing institutional commitment to aging.

In submitting proposals which require matching or cost sharing on the part of the institution, you will need to secure this match from the appropriate person at your institution. At a large university this may be the academic vice president or the vice president for financial affairs. In a smaller setting it may be the academic dean or the president. In any event, if the match is secured, regardless if the proposal is funded, you may argue for the match to be translated into university funds earmarked for aging. This may not be successful because (1) the money for match is probably prebudgeted for all institutional proposals already and is used solely for that purpose, and (2) the match may be largely in-kind contributions with few hard dollars included. However, if the match is secured, it does, perhaps in some small way, commit the institution to the notion of supporting aging programs. If other outside funds are secured in other ways it may be possible to argue that the ratio or percentage of outside funds to university funds has created an unhealthy balance in your program, therefore more university funds are required.

3. *Academic Legitimacy.* Let's look at the third problem I mentioned, that of academic legitimacy. There are plenty of reference works available regarding different organizational models which can be used to develop a degree or specialization in gerontology.

On the one hand it may be desirable to have substantial autonomy, separate budgets, and an identity which is not too closely aligned with any single discipline or degree program. On the other hand, too much autonomy tends to diffuse one's image and make you impotent with the administration and with your colleagues. Multidisciplinary efforts require a considerable amount of energy if your program thrust is to go beyond a single department. To include other departments, your multidisciplinary program becomes more of a balancing act to keep disparate constituencies happy. This becomes even more of a balancing act when you're offering off-campus training and service activities. If you're providing technical assistance to social service agencies, you increase your range of constituencies and therefore find yourself becoming more and more stretched out.

In addition, the development of new centers, bureaus, and so forth in gerontology has meant a moving away from the traditional academic model. Even when developing new concentration or degree programs in gerontology within existing departments, problems of legitimizing the program remain. Gerontology does not have the trappings of academe complete with large numbers of separate degree programs, traditions, senior scholars, and a large national professional audience. It has a relatively short history, a theoretical base that can only be described as emerging, and a role that can only be defined as being unclear and somewhat diffused in the university. As a gerontologist, I am quite aware that gerontology is not institutionalized in the academic setting nor is there a single institutionalized model. A certain degree of institutionalization appears necessary even if your goal is to develop a university-wide or multidisciplinary approach. Early identification with an existing degree program is perhaps necessary in order for gerontology to be recognized as a legitimate area of study. Later, an organized phasing in of gerontology with other programs is possible when an acceptable identity for gerontology has been established. Attempts on the part of individuals not to become institutionalized may lead to gerontology programs being carved up by academic entrepreneurs and fiscal budget cutters.

3. External Considerations (Nonacademic)

In developing programs in gerontology, it is important to know your institution, to know its "mission" and its natural student market. All of us can lay claim to a certain natural market. Urban universities may develop programs focusing on urban problems/opportunities such as mass transit, crime and victimization, density and urban relocation problems, and so forth. Rural institutions may emphasize population loss, physical isolation, or transportation problems. If you live in an area where an ethnic or minority group is predominant, this may become a program focus and so forth. There is then a certain natural constituency and a natural market for an institution of higher education.

Sometimes this mission is not well understood. I recall an experience a few years ago when I was teaching at a small state college in southern West Virginia in the heart of the Appalachians. We had a student body of some 2,000 students located in a small town of slightly over 1,000 people. We were surrounded by coal mines, small farms, and a heavily dependent population characterized by high rates of various social and medical pathologies. Being fresh out of graduate school, I and others decided to develop a degree program in urban studies! In retrospect, the notion was absurd. We had few faculty and monetary resources, certainly no urban area. Fortunately, wiser heads prevailed and the program was not developed.

It is important to have some idea of the kind of students that would be attracted to your institution and to your program. Are they young or old, graduate or undergraduate, experienced or inexperienced? The best plan of attack is probably to orient the program to satisfy the largest single block of students. We know the history of gerontology is such that few academic programs were available in the United States until quite recently. At the present time, there are many sections of the country where little or no graduate or undergraduate education is available in gerontology. In our case we have some 200 students taking off-campus courses in five different locations around the state. Over 90 percent of those 200 students are made up of agency personnel who work for the departments of welfare, social security, mental health, and so forth. As a result, our largest constituency consists of state agency personnel.

Periodically it is desirable to review institutional access to both on-campus and off-campus training facilities. The national figures on the adult as a learner are readily available. What are too often ignored are the possibilities for involvement with consortiums or with other universities for cross listing of courses and the sharing of faculty. Other program options may include external degrees, correspondence courses, continuing education, university without walls, weekend colleges, night schools, minimesters, and interim terms. In order to be responsive to off-campus needs, courses may need to be repackaged in a manner that is substantially different from that in the traditional academic mode.

4. Developing Gerontology Programs

Lastly, a few comments about the organization of gerontology programs. Decisions about the future development of gerontology programs are often made unintentionally early when the program is first begun. Decisions about degree versus concentration, single versus multidisciplinary efforts, personnel, and financial support are often made in response to larger university or governmental demands. I would argue that it is not merely desirable, but imperative that emerging programs consciously determine their own program thrust. The thrust may be more applied and involve the practice professions such as social work, nursing, counseling, home economics, public administration, or regional planning. It may be more traditionally academic such as that found in sociology, psychology, political science, or economics. Or, it may be a blend of the two. Regardless, either the motivation of money from external sources and its concomitant restrictions or existing academic structures may so quickly determine a program's thrust that program originators are never really quite sure how their program developed as it did.

Perhaps the second major decision is whether to go the single degree route in gerontology versus the program option or concentration. I would strongly suggest the latter even though this is, admittedly, a minority position in the nation. My reasons are:

1. A degree is insufficient and narrow training in a field where the broadest exposure to other disciplines and knowledge areas is desirable.

2. A degree limits job/career options to more strictly "aging" positions rather than to more general positions of social worker, sociologist, or psychologist with training in aging.

3. A degree program amounts to additional competition for scarce university resources.

4. A degree cannot be certified at the present time as no national or regional accreditation boards exist in gerontology. As a result, considerable variation exists in degree programs with resultant confusion as to their meaning.

5. A degree is philosophically inconsistent with the meaning of "gerontology" as it has traditionally meant a more eclectic approach.

6. A degree reduces campus options for expansion at the doctoral and master's level and into other departments and academic areas. It becomes difficult to develop true interdisciplinary relationships because gerontology as a degree program becomes the "property" of one department or division.

Reference

Ikenberry, S. O., and Freidman, R. C. *Beyond academic departments*. San Francisco: Jossey-Bass, 1972.

Section Two
Curriculum Development

Some of the specifics of course development were discussed in the preconference workshops. The papers from those workshops can be found in the appendix. In this section the papers deal with the broader aspects of curriculum issues, including both resources for obtaining information and program models that range in complexity from single-discipline models to consortia in gerontology.

The last three papers of this section examine important dimensions of three types of curricular organizations for teaching and research in gerontology. They focus on examples of programs in gerontology: first, the "single-disciplinary" program, then the multi- and interdisciplinary format, and third, the consortium arrangement involving several colleges and universities. The authors did not intend merely to describe the efforts with which they were familiar—they were not simply engaging in show-and-tell. They have attempted to derive some principles of operations from their own respective activities—to identify concepts that pertain to *our* experience and points of view.

The order of topics is presumably from simple to complex: initially, a single-discipline curriculum with gerontology as a major; secondly, the aspects of multi- and interdisciplinary programs at a large university with some history of gerontological involvement; and finally, at perhaps the most complex level of organization, the involvement in a multi-institutional consortium.

Curriculum Materials in Gerontology

Margaret E. Hartford
University of Southern California

The title of this workshop is Curriculum Materials in Gerontology. The following people have contributed to the development of the content: Dr. Richard Davis, Director of Publications of the Andrus Gerontology Center; Ms. Emily Miller, Librarian of the Andrus Center Research and Reference Library; Dr. Anthony Lenzer, Director of the Gerontology Institute, University of Hawaii; Ms. Carol Van Steenberg and Robin Karasik of the KWIC Training Resources in Aging Project of the Duke University Center for the Study of Aging and Human Development.

When we speak of curriculum in gerontology, we may be referring to many kinds of programs, courses, student groups, settings, or institutions and educational objectives. All have in common, at an abstract level, the improvement of the quality of life of older people. The immediate student group may be the general public, children from preschool through high school, undergraduates, young adults, middle aged, and older adults themselves. The context of the curriculum may be popular, through educational or commercial media T.V. and radio, or public lecture series, content in the educational system K through 12, the community college or adult school, university undergraduate or graduate programs, professional school with gerontology specialties, or gerontology courses related to professional specialties.

Curriculum in gerontology means many things to different people. We may refer to content on aging submerged within a general course on human behavior, social policy, social, economic, or political theory, physical development and change, or social philosophy. Or, on the other hand, there may be specific courses on aging, such as Fundamentals of Gerontology or Issues and Concepts in Aging, taught as an overview for the public, or for undergraduates and the uncommitted graduates. There are even more specifics: Sociology of Aging, Social Policy in Aging, Psychology of Aging, Physiology of Aging, the practice courses of working with older adults in nursing, in the human services, in adult education, in social work, in public administration, in law. Or topical courses such as Emotional Problems of Aging, Sex after Sixty, Aging Parents and Their Off-Spring, Preretirement Planning and Education. There are now literally hundreds of courses in gerontology in every possible curricular arrangement, including the Sunrise Semester for the early morning eager learners.

To look at it another way, then, when we consider curriculum in gerontology we may be considering (1) education of the general public about older people (ranging from children to the older people themselves) and dealing with knowledge, and particularly with attitudes, (2) preretirement education—in the middle years, which should start early in life and no later than entry into the job market, (3) senior adult education, activity for engagement, creativity, enhancement, survival, continuity in relationships, (4) higher education for scholarship, research, knowledge, and knowledge building, and (5) career education or preparation for professional practice with and in behalf of older adults in such specific areas as health services, law, social services, religious practice, housing and environment planning, public administration where there is emphasis on practice skills, knowledge, attitudes, and application of the findings of scientific research into the real world.

We are considering part of a course, a full course, a sequence of courses, a full curriculum, or an Institute or School of Gerontology.

Within this possible framework of curriculum, we are asked to consider resources for curriculum. Some of the others will suggest certain hardware and software instruments. I would like to focus on a few examples of use of students' experiences, of older people themselves as curricular resources, and the use of experiential learning.

The most obvious resource is having a student body, or class composition, covering a wide range of ages. Where possible, it is advantageous to have older people as teaching assistants, class participants, tutors, guest lecturers, or course instructors. We have heard of gerontologists who have never had face-to-face contact with an older person, who have intellectual mastery of a body of content, without ever testing it in a real world. There is the research gerontologist for whom older people are a sample, a statistic, a subject of an interview, totally dehumanized, as Dr. Comfort has referred to in *A Good Age* [New York: Crown, 1976].

Older people, as well as younger ones, need to consider the content of gerontology within the context of being old. Simulations and role playing are helpful tools, experiencing what it feels like—both to have annoying little decrements such as deteriorating vision and hearing, some slowing of pace or of capacity to respond quickly, or the big annoyances which result from catastrophic or chronic illnesses such as arthritis, heart, or respiratory diseases. Empathy and identification can begin through simulation, but it becomes more real if there is day-to-day interaction through collegial study together, field experiences, interviewing, or listening carefully.

Do you remember the Peanuts cartoon a few months ago, when Lucy was writing the essay about her grandmother, and she ended by saying, "and after World War II, grandmother left her job in the defense plant, and went to work at the telephone company, we need to study the lives of great women like my grandmother. . . . so talk to your grandmother, you may discover that she has more interesting talents than baking peanut butter cookies." So talk with older people. Students in many classes have made use of taped interviews with older people at home, in the park, in nursing homes, in nutrition programs, on buses, not for exploitation, but for enriching experiences.

A retired social worker friend of mine, who left a New York City national staff job, went to live in the mountains of Pennsylvania. During the bicentennial year she and an adult education group of hers undertook to prepare a slide and tape show of interviews with very old people who still pursued crafts and arts and skills. The project, which took a year of seeking out people to be interviewed, conducting the interviews and taking pictures, included a 100-year-old accordian player in a sing-along with his family, family coal mining related by a 92-year-old, flax spinning by an 82-year-old woman, and several other skills by similarly aged persons, such as making quilts, building log cabins, making wagons, producing and spinning wool, weaving, and rug making. Both the project and the product are good resources for curriculum for persons of all ages, and have applicability for psychology of aging, sociology of aging, and senior adult education, among other areas.

Another type of project, and one many of us have used is "design your own bibliography" or "design your own textbook." Although the literature in gerontology is expanding and more textbooks are becoming available, there still are not adequate texts in some areas. One project, therefore, is to have students choose topics reflecting their own interests and then search the literature for relevant articles. This search is extended not only to technical journals in the biological and social sciences, in the professions, in gerontology and geriatrics, but in popular magazines or in far out, seemingly unrelated materials. Such a search may alert students to research and existing knowledge they did not know existed, or to the lack of it as well as the need for research or articles to be prepared for publication. As they abstract and critique articles they construct a bibliography for themselves and their classmates.

One of my introductory classes, two years ago, was distressed because there was not an introductory text that was useful for the course. As part of the final exam, they were asked to outline a text that would be appropriate for the course, and then to select one topical chapter and discuss the content that should be included. The latter part was drawn from course projects each had done in which the student had reviewed a particular kind of need or resource for the elderly. The net result of their answers was the outline of a text which a publisher has taken, and the engagement of professionals or educators to develop the chapters from their specialized knowledge and experience. This is where social gerontology is at this time.

Building genealogies, local histories, topical interests in antiques and old things of value, begins a sensitivity for preretired young and middle-aged people. Reminiscence helps older people find a sense of value and integrity and meaning, if done well. Both involve people in interaction with each other in a real world that works not only on knowledge but stereotypes, attitudes, and values.

These are only examples to stimulate some thinking about using or developing curricular resources.

KWIC: A Developing Information Service
for Training in Aging

Carol L. Van Steenberg
Western Gerontological Society
Robin B. Karasik
Duke University

Millions of dollars are being expended annually to develop curricular materials for training in aging.[1] Yet, until quite recently, very little provision has been made for evaluating such materials, revising them, or disseminating them. Typically, materials simply are developed, used by the trainer(s) responsible for delivering the particular training event, and—costs permitting—distributed to *one* round of trainees. The materials are then usually forgotten. Under such circumstances there can be little hope for improvement in the state of the art, since there is little accumulation and refinement of experience. Each trainer or educator begins from "ground zero," does what he or she can, and usually has little impact on the field. This wastefulness of creative energy is unfortunate, at best; in a time of increasing demand for training in aging at all levels, it is a great misfortune.

To conserve creative efforts in gerontology materials development and to link trainers in the field of aging with the resources they need but often cannot obtain, the Duke Center for the Study of Aging and Human Development KWIC Training Resources in Aging Project has been developed over the past two years.[2] (The KWIC Project's full name is "Key Word Indexed Collection of Training Resources in Aging Project.") With a long-range goal of improving training in the field of aging, the KWIC Project has as its intermediate objectives developing and providing various supportive services to designers and deliverers of training in aging.

The purpose of this paper is three-fold:

1. To provide a brief developmental history of the KWIC project
2. To identify and address some of the conceptual and practical issues inherent in developing an information resource useable by and useful to academics and practitioners in aging
3. To describe KWIC's response to these issues, i.e., its design, operations, products, and services

Historical Perspective

In 1973 the Duke Center began two related aging training projects under funding from the Administration on Aging (Older Americans Act, Title IV-A): one, a broad-gauged educational modeling effort to focus on the design and implementation of models for delivering training in aging; the other, a specific short-term training project aimed at ACTION's Older Americans Volunteer Programs' Project Directors. With the initiation of these projects, an attempt was made to identify relevant training materials others had produced and to learn from their experience. It soon became clear that training in aging was characterized by extreme fragmentation and that training materials were ephemeral, rarely evaluated, infrequently collected, and virtually never categorized or catalogued in an accessible manner. In short, chaos reigned and it seemed rather pointless to develop more materials which soon would be lost, unless some effort was begun to capture and systematize such resources.

Accordingly, contact was made with the nine other short-term training projects funded by the Administration on Aging. They were asked to share curricula they were using, any additions or adaptations devised during the training process (all were training multiple sets of trainees), and any evaluative data collected as to the effectiveness of such training materials. Because of their cooperation, more was salvaged from that series of experiences than from any previous venture in aging training.

A search then was begun for a method of organizing both the Duke Center's training experience and its emerging collection of materials. No single, conventional approach could be identified so an eclectic, pragmatic approach was forged. *Social planning* provided a systems approach (encompassing evaluation); *community organization* helped in conceptualizing accessing problems and suggesting solutions (outreach, needs assessment, network development); *educational technology* focused attention on the instructional process within a systematic framework; and *information sciences* provided both an apt acronymic name for the project and a means to begin accessing the collection—key word indexing—which did not mandate premature categorization.

Besides the pursuit of ephemeral materials, a number of activities were initiated in line with these approaches during KWIC's first year of operation. Aimed at increasing both the information available about training materials in aging and the sophistication of the typical seeker of information, these activities included:

1. The development of an audiovisual evaluation instrument focusing on key instructional elements
2. A "Film Festival" procedure to review and evaluate selected films in the new collection of training materials
3. A one-day workshop on systematic instruction to address the skills needed in developing health-related educational materials in aging
4. The production of the first edition of the *Keyword Index to Training Resources in Aging*
5. The publication of a monthly *Library Newsletter*
6. The initiation of "Film Forum," reporting the evaluation of selected audiovisuals

KWIC Project Design

These efforts demonstrated the utility and necessity for a mixed but coordinated approach. In 1975 a concentrated effort to collect, categorize, evaluate, and provide information about training resources in aging was begun. This effort came to be known as the "KWIC Training Resources in Aging Project" or KWIC.

Although KWIC's initial focus was narrow (assembling and sharing evaluated short-term training materials), strong and unanticipated demands from long-term trainers rapidly necessitated a broadening of focus. KWIC's intention was defined: KWIC was eventually to be an easily accessed system comprised of *evaluated* training materials for every audience and every educational objective relevant to the field of aging. Because responsiveness to the emerging information needs of trainers and educators in the multidisciplinary field of aging was to be the crucial factor guiding the system's development, flexibility as a characteristic of the system was presupposed. Further, precedence was given to developing communications mechanisms adequate for:

1. Conveying to KWIC what its "clients" needed in the short run (both as individuals and as a group) and in the long run
2. Conveying to KWIC information about new resources of interest to its clientele
3. Transmitting to KWIC's clients information about what KWIC could and could not do for them
4. Providing feedback to KWIC on the usefulness of given training resources, the utility of particular kinds of information about training resources and, ultimately, the value of KWIC in improving the quality of training in aging

Early data gleaned from KWIC's clients indicated that *any* information about existing training resources was valuable. Thus, an initial emphasis either upon only evaluated resources or upon developing evaluative information could not be justified as "responsive to the emerging information needs of trainers." Because trainers and educators could gain access to research information in gerontology through other avenues, albeit imperfectly, the decision was made to include in the KWIC "system" only resources clearly linked to educational or training experiences. KWIC would not attempt to cover the broader field of aging-related research information but would provide referral to other appropriate information systems, sources, or services.

KWIC Project Operations

The design principles of flexibility and fluid communication have been instrumental in shaping current project operations.

In order to provide KWIC with the information it needs to respond best to inquiries from trainers about resources, KWIC's inquirers are helped to frame their questions efficiently. Trainers are asked to articulate:

1. Who they wish to train (i.e., the level of sophistication of the intended audience)

2. What they intend to accomplish via the training (i.e., content coverage and educational objectives)

3. Other factors of importance in their training (i.e., setting, length)

Not only does this procedure lead to a better "answer" from KWIC but feedback from trainers indicates it is helpful in conceptualizing the training task. The majority of the requests for KWIC services have been from:

1. University-based aging programs
2. Local social service or public human service agencies
3. State units on aging
4. Long-term care facilities
5. Consulting organizations
6. Students

The major kinds of information demanded by users have been in the following areas:

1. General information on aging
2. General information on audiovisual resources in aging
3. Materials for long-term care training/education
4. Educational programs for the elderly
5. Aging course outlines or curricula
6. Materials to develop counseling skills

Geographically, KWIC's users are concentrated in the United States, with some international inquiries.

The "information base" upon which KWIC draws consists primarily of materials which have been collected, screened, coded, and indexed. Such materials are not only cited in the *Keyword Index to Training Resources in Aging*, but are accessible to KWIC staff and others to examine or reproduce if necessary. New candidates for inclusion are sought continuously and are received daily. The methods employed to acquire likely resources include regular searches of relevant on-line data bases (e.g., ERIC, MEDLINE, CATLINE, NTIS, etc.), scanning of approximately 25 journals and newsletters monthly and, most importantly, directly contacting likely producers of materials (e.g., recipients of Older Americans Act Title IV-A funds).

Information dissemination activities are vigorously pursued to inform trainers and educators about KWIC's capacity to provide assistance in resource identification and selection. Distributing project descriptions, submitting letters to the editors of relevant journals, making presentations at national and state meetings of trainers are but three examples of these activities.

KWIC Project Services and Products

The KWIC project provides a variety of services and products to trainers and educators:

1. *The Keyword Index to Training Resources in Aging*, produced semiannually, is available in both microfilm and print editions. The *Index* is divided into two sections: (a) a listing of resources arranged by broad categories and (b) a display of these resources by keywords. Detailed information explaining the *Index*'s use for selecting resources precedes both listings.

2. *Individually tailored resource lists* are developed in response to requests from trainers.

3. *Consultation on resource selection* is provided to trainers seeking assistance.

4. *Consultation on training design is given* on a limited basis. At present this is available at KWIC by appointment.

5. *Film Forum*, reporting evaluations of selected audiovisuals, is published three times a year. Its film profiles are based on data from professional and nonprofessional users of audiovisuals and include information on subject matter, perceived purpose, recommended audiences, suggested use, and an overall rating.

6. *Library Newsletter: Information Resources in Gerontology*, which alerts researchers to aging references other than those found in standard gerontological journals, is published monthly. Special features include selected annotated bibliographies and reviews of training resources.

The "individually tailored resource list" is the service most frequently provided by KWIC, although this is often combined with providing "consultation on resource selection."

KWIC staff, in answering requests, use a number of tools, two of which are listed above, *The Keyword Index to Training Resources in Aging*, and the *Film Forum*. Both of these are available at the cost of their duplication (or printing) and mailing. While these tools enable a trainer/educator to identify a significant portion of the resources which KWIC has acquired, KWIC staff may be contacted directly to determine if relevant new resources have been identified. KWIC staff also maintains, for referral purposes, a resource file of pertinent information which cannot be *Index*ed, e.g., names of experts, documents that are not linked specifically to education/training, and listings of information sources/services.

The KWIC Project receives inquiries by mail, telephone, and in person. For clarity, each inquiry is analyzed to determine the classes of resources likely to be useful, i.e., the *level of sophistication of the intended audience* (students or trainees), the *subject matter* (educational objectives) to be addressed, and the *extent of information desired* by the inquirer about resources (e.g., is he/she seeking others' course outlines? seeking references to texts that could be used? seeking help in developing the objectives of the course?). In making this assessment of the inquirer's information needs, KWIC staff may need to recontact the inquirer, by mail or telephone, for clarification.

Once the inquirer's needs are determined, the "search" begins. First, KWIC staff select categories and keywords which are likely to access resources addressing the inquirer's needs. Because the keywords used to access the resources are limited, it is much more helpful for KWIC staff to have the training information outlined above rather than the inquirer's own suggested keywords. If the inquirer's key word(s) do not match KWIC's, KWIC staff will have to make a guess on the best match. Both the *Index* and the new, not yet indexed, resources are searched—*manually*—by KWIC staff utilizing the categories and keywords selected. Generally this procedure yields a number of candidates which then are examined. If these prove, on inspection, to be of likely use with respect to the training task defined by the inquirer, they are included in the individually tailored list of resources KWIC provides.

In the rare event that no relevant resources are found in this pool, KWIC staff check an "ancillary" resource file containing materials and sources KWIC has collected which cannot be *Index*ed (e.g., workshop announcements, program descriptions, course lists without content elaboration, etc.). Should some of these address the inquirer's question, he or she would be informed of these, particularly where a contact person can be identified from whom to seek additional information. If the question posed was not strictly a "KWIC" question, i.e., did not address education or training and aging, the inquirer would be referred to other sources of information (e.g., if it were a research question, to standard library sources and appropriate on-line data bases). More importantly, if the question was clearly an aging-training/education inquiry, yet could not be "answered" with the resources at KWIC's disposal, KWIC staff would take note of this information gap and would intensify their efforts to obtain materials in this area.

Research and Development Activities

One of the major stumbling blocks KWIC has faced is trying to build a system from materials which have not been developed "systematically." Such materials may be good and useful, but it is not easy to tell how good they are or for whom they are good. Thus KWIC has had the task of developing methods by which information can be collected for trainers about the "instructional potential" of the training resources held by KWIC. Two strategies have been developed.

The first strategy is known as "screening" and is done by KWIC project staff. Each training document is examined and a notation is made (i.e., it is coded) to indicate the presence in the document of the following elements of the systematic approach to instruction: purpose (or rationale), audience, stated objectives, instructional strategies, evaluation instruments (methodology), and evaluation data.

This procedure does not provide direct *qualitative* information about a document; it only tells the user how "complete" a given resource is. Thus, an apparently very complete document may have objectives which are unreasonable and unmeasurable, an audience which is ill-defined and an evaluation report which is meaningless. However, it is much more frequently the case that when the elements of systematic instruction have been considered and addressed by a materials producer, a better resource is the result.

To attack the "quality" problem more directly, another strategy is being pursued. Key resources in the KWIC system are to be analyzed from both a "content validity" and an "educational methodology" perspective. Applying a methodology to analyze materials' instructional design will enable the assessment of the likely value and effectiveness of training resources in given settings. Current plans point to the completion of such analyses for one subset of KWIC resources by April 1977. This will provide the test of the instrument adapted for this purpose and may result in its refinement.

In summary, KWIC is an information system, in its developmental phase, which is designed to provide service to planners of training in aging. The KWIC Project is ambitious in its attempt to attend to the problems of evaluative research, cope with the multidisciplinary field of gerontology, address the issues posed by the educational process, and accomplish this in a manner that is appealing and useful to those faced with delivering educational programs in gerontology or to older people. Since its inception, the KWIC project has been self-consciously as systematic as possible in its efforts to accumulate and transmit knowledge about resources. Its methodology has been eclectic, with several approaches relevant to KWIC's design and implementation: social planning (including evaluation), community organization, educational technology, and information sciences. Its ultimate purpose— improving the quality of training in the field of aging—can only be accomplished with the cooperation of the users.

Notes

1. In fiscal year 1976 and the transition period covering July–October, 1976, the Administration on Aging awarded $14 million under Title IV-A of the Older Americans Act. (In *Aging*, Dec. 1976–Jan. 1977, p. 8.)

2. The KWIC Training Resources in Aging Project is supported by Grant 94-P-20384-04 DHEW, OHD, AoA, Title IV-A.

Gerontology—A Single-Discipline Model

Anne M. McIver
Molloy College

The case for the need of studies and programs in the field of gerontology has been well documented. But the implementation of the foregoing has left much to be desired. We have been exposed both to some well-devised programs, as well as those that were dangling and fragmented.

At Molloy College we met the challenge of a concentration in gerontology by proposing and now implementing a B.A. degree program. Basically we present gerontology as a single discipline, taking its place equally with other existing disciplines on the campus. This program was approved by New York State's Department of Higher Education.

Our strongest defense for the single-discipline approval was to prevent the dilution and loss of impact that gerontology would suffer if treated simply as additional courses distributed among the other disciplines. Presenting a structured and cohesive approach that gave gerontology its proper import, we concluded, was the only way to protect the training, education, and research needed in this field.

The major in gerontology is designed to provide a study of the physiological, psychological, and sociological aspects of the process of aging.

Its primary purpose is to offer the student training both in general and specific areas in gerontology. The student is enabled to have an entry level opportunity in the field as well as a basis for advanced studies.

Molloy's concern with the challenge presented by our aging population stems from its belief in the dignity and worth of each individual.

Before embarking on the new program an exhaustive survey should be done to ascertain the "needs" of the surrounding communities and the "opportunities" that would be afforded to graduates. The resulting program must be an expression of the particular college and relative to its internal structure. The objectives of a program in gerontology should include:

A. To enlighten students as to the services they can render by careers in gerontology
B. To promulgate the following objectives for the gerontology major:
   1. Recognition and acceptance within their own personality of the normal facets of aging. *Indicated by*:
      a. Acceptance of aging as a natural phenomenon with positive attitudes toward this process
      b. Acceptance of death and dying as a part of living, making them capable of coping with the idea of death for themselves and others
   2. Effective communication of the positive composites of aging. *Indicated by*:
      a. Ability to inspire a feeling of concern for the elderly
      b. Maintenance of good working relationships with the elderly which will help them to reach their ultimate potential
      c. Ability to establish fruitful communication with all persons in any way associated with the life of the aging
   3. Understanding of milieu therapy especially in the area of long-term care. *Indicated by*:
      a. Commitment to and participation in a program in which the aging are assessed, evaluated, and programmed to realize their optimum potential
      b. Respect for the aged as individuals who have dignity and the right to:
         1) Privacy
         2) Use of time
         3) Personal property
         4) Choice of activities
         5) Independence
      c. Rendering help to the elderly person so he/she may be able to perform well in situations involving:
         1) Rights of others
         2) Group process
         3) Group decision
         4) Friendship
         5) Communication

      d. Knowledge of the effective use of the tools of therapy:
          1) Art
          2) Music
          3) Poetry, etc.
      e. Ability to help the elderly reach a clarification of a "value hierarchy"
      f. Understanding of and ability to deal with unacceptable behavior
      g. Maintenance of a warm and accepting environment
  4. Manifestation of the use of practical means to attain the goals of working with the elderly. *Indicated by:*
      a. Wise selection and use of a variety of media
      b. Use of variety of media to stimulate creativity
      c. Encouragement of the aged to participate in appropriate programs
      d. Adapting materials and methods to the abilities of the aged
      e. Awareness and use of a variety of techniques to assess all and different aspects of aged in various programs
  5. Acceptance of self-evaluation. *Indicated by:*
      a. Willingness to seek critical feedback
      b. Evidence of seeking to expand knowledge in the field of gerontology:
          1) Participation/attendance at conferences, workshops, in-service courses
          2) Matriculation in a graduate program

The program is interdisciplinary. It is supported by every department in the college.

All students must fulfill a college core consisting of liberal arts subjects and a discipline core. A total of 128 credits is required for graduation.

Gerontology majors program—B.A. degree

College core requirements	49
Major requirements	45
Electives (under consultation with advisor)	34
Total	128

Major requirements	*Credits*
Introduction to Gerontology	3
General Psychology	3
Principles of Biology	3
Biology of Aging	3
Educational Gerontology	3
Economics of Aging	3
Sociology of Aging	3

Nutrition for Geriatrics	3
Recreational Leadership in Gerontology	3
Psychology of Aging	3
Foundations of Thanatology	3
Abnormal Psychology	3
Dynamics of Behavior	3
Practicum	6
Total	45

Keeping in mind variations and a wide margin of flexibility, this model could be implemented in those four-year colleges who are mainly contained in a liberal arts framework. It provides new choices for the student body. Our gerontological model does not detract from existing disciplines because it addresses itself to a target population they left untapped.

Multidisciplinary Programs in Gerontology

Joseph H. Britton
Pennsylvania State University

The Pennsylvania State University has had some 30 years of activity of one kind or another in the field of aging, which effort began with adult education and research on nutritional, economic, and community problems, and on individual and family studies of later maturity and old age. It was natural that those efforts led to course development, to cooperative research, eventually to program development at the graduate and undergraduate levels in a variety of fields. After many years, events have led to a reasonably well-coordinated effort as a university.

As a university, Penn State has been fortunate in having faculty and administrators who recognized the importance of gerontology as a developing field and who saw the wisdom of the resources being used to develop competence in gerontology. While these developments have not been simply luck, and in fact have required plenty of hard work by a number of faculty members, I believe coincidence has also played an important part in our own gerontological history. Many events seem to have happened together in fortunate ways.

Our history has included the availability and use of federal and state funding for special purposes, in addition to honest, hard-money commitments of the University's ongoing resources. Having a decade of funding of research training by the National Institute on Aging and its predecessor institute, nearly a half-decade of funding academician-practitioner training by the Administration on Aging, the funding of a few years' worth of continuing education and community service projects by the State's Office for the Aging, federal funding of various research projects, and most recently of the operational grant for the University's Gerontology Center—all of these have very directly aided program development at Penn State. Although Penn State has built solidly with "hard money" for faculty personnel, in particular, I would be remiss if I did not point out the importance of such material aid to gerontological programs.

These remarks lead me to the first of several statements which I see as principles pertaining to the development of multidisciplinary programs in gerontology. Most of my comments are derived from experience in professional and graduate education, less with undergraduate studies.

1. Programs are organized and implemented within a particular social and historical and political milieu, and often they "grow up" without great logic or forethought about what they might become. Faculty operate within academic contexts at a particular time in their history, in the history of the institution and of the field. They may play a part in choosing among alternatives for individual and institutional investment of time, effort and funding for program development. This reminds us that programs should be viewed as lying in a unique time frame and within a unique social-economic-political context. Change the time, the *dramatis personae*, the political and economic situation, and the outcome will change. While we should try to learn from each other, we should be careful about imitating each other. The new program might well turn out to be far better than the pattern we are following!

2. From my view, gerontology is by definition "multidisciplinary." Therefore, the true gerontologist is a multidisciplinarian, if not an interdisciplinarian. Aging involves changes over time in a variety of domains of behavior, and generally, the domains function together, not separately. Problems of aging do not fall into the confines of the disciplines in spite of how disciplines have been defined by their adherents.

3. It seems equally clear that modern scholarship and the technology of each of the sciences, the arts, and the professions, require deep understanding of particular and often highly specialized areas of knowledge. Acquiring deep knowledge and understanding is impossible on a great front of information and practice. Thus, at the graduate level one must specialize to a considerable degree, by developing focused competence and in order to gain valid respectability within a field or discipline. Therefore, gerontological training and research efforts should be carried out in the separate disciplinary-bound programs. Among the best gerontologists will be those well-grounded in specialized fields in which specialists apply their particular techniques of scholarship to processes and problems of aging.

4. Again, without disagreeing with myself, I do explicitly include the need for *interdisciplinary* programs which focus efforts on aging within a prescribed subject matter domain, and such programs can take their place

alongside discipline-bound or professionally specific programs. At Penn State, we have both multi- and interdisciplinary programs. The major interdisciplinary program took on a life-span perspective, but this was the location of primary administrative and faculty commitment to gerontology. Still the time resources were very limited and many other areas competed for their "place in the sun."

However, the particular gerontologists who gathered on the scene wanted to promote the incorporation of aging into already-established programs rather than to compete with them. This was a deliberate political strategy to gain cooperation, for to make a program go we needed all the gerontologists we could muster. Our first training fund application was initiated by three faculty in three departments. To ensure our viability we needed all three and all of the resources and status together that we could muster to make gerontology endeavors strong and academically respectable within the institution.

Thus, in our case, we have a number of graduate majors in which it is possible to emphasize gerontology. We do not have a gerontology major per se nor do I perceive any move to create one.

5. In multidisciplinary and interdisciplinary programs, special efforts need to be made to make opportunities for students to come together for academic and professional socialization. In the form of colloquia, field trips, etc., these efforts have considerable significance for developing basic understanding of gerontology as a field.

6. For many reasons, programs need the interest and support of advisers outside the university, and care is needed in selection of such advisers and defining their roles and using their advice. They should help relate programs to the community and help enable service programs to take advantage of the resources of the university.

7. Aging as a process is best seen in reference to a continuum of processes of growing up, maturing, and growing old. The same can be said of programs of training professional or preprofessional persons for working with the elderly. This is not to say, however, that professional knowledge and competence are entirely generic and can be transferred with ease from one client population to another. It is to claim that aging can best be seen in reference to continuity and change over the life span.

8. I want to make a few comments about the program with which I personally have been identified: Penn State's program in *human development and family studies*. This program "focuses on the interdisciplinary, developmental study of individuals, small groups, and families—for the purpose of expanding basic knowledge and improving professional application." One area of emphasis in this interdisciplinary program is *adult development and aging*, from postadolescence through maturity and old age. It concerns also the contexts of such change and professional programs for dealing with problems of the middle and later years. The overall program usually has about 100 students in residence and a faculty of 35 or 40 persons. I note some of its

features and some of the problems and prospects in operating it:

a. There will probably always be a discrepancy between the ideal program, as defined in the descriptive material and the stated aspirations, and the program as it actually functions.

b. Gerontological subject matter must compete for its share of internal resources and status along with all other areas.

c. Conversely, being funded more generously by outside funds than some other areas, gerontologists must also make certain their special resources benefit the total program; usually this will be indirect help. This requires administrative and faculty efforts to develop the total program which will flourish only if its parts serve the whole.

d. An interdisciplinary program in a university should build upon the basic disciplines and the courses those departments offer rather than trying to replace those basic courses with their own. This is the economic way for the program to operate, of course. The special mission of inter- and multidisciplinary programs is to put such information *together*. We try to do this by elaboration of the knowledge base, by devising programs of intervention, and by testing such programs in the field and applying those to familial or community settings.

e. There must be an adequate research base for graduate programs to sustain their own teaching and service programs, but a variety of types of projects should be encouraged. This has obvious benefit for students and faculty and should be a source of renewal of knowledge.

f. Likewise, there should be a variety of ties to professional practitioner settings and to community agencies and policy systems operating *in vivo*. These ties should also serve to relate teaching and research to the fundamental problems of functioning individuals, families, and communities. Further, such ties help to provide practicum opportunities for students.

g. Programs should be flexibly designed to build upon students' knowledge and experience, but advisers must accept their responsibility to define and insist upon competence in the important domains.

h. We should continue to aspire to achieve excellence in multidisciplinary and interdisciplinary teaching and research, and we should be honest in our evaluation of all such programs.

9. In the inter- and multidisciplinary contexts in which I have experience, I see a number of continuing problems and difficulties. They may be obvious to all, so I shall list them without much comment:

a. The balance between breadth and depth in subject matter coverage: The greatest danger of our program is superficiality.

b. The difficulty of a diverse faculty arriving at a consensus of what the *essentials* of a heterogeneous interdisciplinary program really are.

c. The difficulty of recruiting and maintaining a diverse and heterogeneous faculty which will work together in carrying out the program objectives.

d. The problem of perceived status and financial differentials between and among persons identified with different disciplines or fields, among practitioners and theoreticians.

e. The obtaining and making available the resources to stimulate and maintain programmatic efforts in a variety of fields.

f. The problem of defining priorities for program development, directions which show respect for the program objectives as well as for the desires of individual faculty to develop their own specialties.

g. The problem of resisting the temptation to delay or to divert program priorities and program resources, and to extend staff unwisely, solely on the basis of "soft-money" support.

h. The problem of assuring that we have leaders who see, foresee, and proclaim horizons and potentials of multi- and interdisciplinary programmatic efforts.

Consortia in Gerontology

Melvin A. White
University of Utah

A consortium is an arrangement whereby three or more educational institutions formally join forces to achieve a common educational goal.

By the mid-sixties, it was possible for Raymond Moore to identify 1,017 formal cooperative arrangements in American higher education in which more than 1,500 institutions were participating (Moore, 1968).

In 1970, Lewis D. Patterson undertook a more discriminating inventory, concentrating on consortia that had some communality because they met similar standards. Thirty-one consortia were identified in meeting five specific requirements: (1) a voluntary formal organization, (2) three or more member institutions, (3) multiacademic programs, (4) at least one full-time professional to administer consortium programs, (5) a required annual contribution or some other tangible evidence of the long-term commitment of member institutions.

Consortia in gerontology are of more recent origin. In 1968, the University of Oregon and Portland State developed an interuniversity gerontology program. Oregon State later joined with the consortium to create a triumvirate.

In 1972, the Rocky Mountain Gerontology Center, which includes Brigham Young University, Southern Utah State College, Utah State University, the University of Utah, and Weber State College was established.

From 1971–1977 an increasing number of gerontology consortium arrangements developed in the United States. The organizational structures and functions of these consortia vary considerably. In reality, most so-called consortium arrangements are little more than working agreements between institutions of higher education.

To differentiate between interuniversity/college cooperative efforts and a consortium requires a more definitive statement of a consortium. For the purpose of this paper, a consortium has, in addition to interinstitutional cooperation, the following characteristics:

1. Three or more institutions of higher education are members.

2. A formal organizational structure exists which allows for the carrying out of planning, organizing, and implementing programs across the consortium.

3. There is at least one full-time professional person assigned to administer the consortium programs.

4. Each institution at the highest administrative level must voluntarily commit their institution to the consortium and make available resources to support the consortium effort.

Most, if not all, current consortium arrangements in gerontology are multidisciplinary in nature. Administrative units on each campus may be housed within a single discipline, but the operational phases usually involve a multiplicity of disciplines.

Rationale for Consortia

Historically, institutions of higher education developed along singular academic lines; departments, reflecting a unitary disciplinary approach were established and continue to be the most common form of intrainstitutional organization.

The grouping of disciplines with common interests and interrelationships into colleges provided the opportunity for interdisciplinary involvement, but departments continued as the basic unit and interdisciplinary efforts remained somewhat limited.

Professional schools, which tend to be eclectic in their knowledge base, have contributed to the expansion of interdisciplinary efforts by utilizing theories, concepts, and principles of several academic disciplines and encouraging students to take courses across departmental lines.

A growing awareness of the multiplicity of causation of social problems and the complexity of all forms of animate and inanimate objects has encouraged academicians and professionals to join together in their search for understanding and knowledge.

Current problems, including the lack of adequate funding, loss of student enrollment, and decreasing public support to institutions of higher education, have resulted in efforts to better utilize existing resources and through so doing, to improve educational and research programs in our universities and colleges. The consortium concept is one such attempt to achieve the latter objective.

The Consortia Controversy

Advocates of consortia state that such arrangements can:

1. Increase the quality of education and research
2. Foster cooperative arrangements thus avoiding unnecessary duplication and conflict
3. Decrease the cost of program operation
4. Increase chances of obtaining federal, state, and private funds
5. Strengthen the programs of smaller institutions by making the resources of the larger institutions available to them

Patterson suggests two fundamental questions which consortia advocates must address themselves to: (1) Is there sufficient promise in existing consortia to justify a belief that they can be made adequately effective; and (2) what are the most practical ways to make the movement really move?

Characteristics of Successful Consortia

A review of the literature reveals some insight into those characteristics that contribute to a successful consortium arrangement:

1. Not less than three, nor more than seven or eight members of the consortium. Some consortia in the United States include as many as 20 members, frequently cutting across the political boundaries of several states. Cooperation requires compromise to be effective. Institutions must be willing to forego achieving their own immediate objectives in favor of objectives that will benefit the consortium as a whole. The larger the number of institutions involved, the less the chances for arriving at acceptable decisions that result in a meaningful product. The possibility of agreement on meaningful issues is not only complicated by the number of institutions involved, but by the diversity and complexity of institutional and state policies under which an institution must function.

A consortium that is small faces different but no less serious problems. Withdrawal of any large member immediately jeopardizes the total operation. A large institution likewise can easily control and manipulate a consortium to its own advantage—which may not be in the interest of other members.

2. A second characteristic of a successful consortium is that they have clear-cut, agreed-upon goals and functions. Included under this characteristic is an understanding and support of the roles assigned to the consortium professional staff as they relate to established goals or objectives.

3. The third characteristic is the availability of a formalized vehicle through which each member of the consortium has the equal opportunity for input in determining consortium policy and implementation of that policy. The same vehicle would be available for resolving conflict or differences among members of the consortium.

4. A fourth characteristic is the total commitment of administration and key faculty to the consortium concept and the goals and objectives of the consortium. The current commitment of many institutional leaders and faculty is toward institutional autonomy and not institutional cooperation.

5. The fifth characteristic of successful consortia is adequate and stable funding for staff and program operation. Most of the consortia in gerontology in the United States today are heavily dependent upon federal funds for their survival. The present policies of those funding agencies do not provide the stability for long-range consortium development. State funds, during this time of tight budgets, are difficult to obtain in sufficient quantity to support consortium operations which must compete with established departments in the institutions.

6. The final characteristic essential to success of a consortium is the executive director. There are no formal guidelines available to use in selecting or training "successful executives." A review of present consortia directors indicates that they have similar characteristics (Patterson). Most tend to be in their 40's and 50's. Their educational backgrounds tend to be in the humanities.

One of the primary roles of the executive director is to be able to mobilize and support cooperative efforts across disciplines and institutions. Observation of higher education leads one to the conclusion that the cooperation between disciplines and institutions seldom develops as a matter of evolution.

A Consortium Model

Currently there exists no one "ideal" consortium model in gerontology. As previously indicated, one of our greatest challenges is to develop an effective working model that will be instrumental in achieving all or most of the advantages of a consortium. In all probability, there never will be a model that fits all occasions. The Rocky Mountain Gerontology Center out of five years of experience developed a model which may be of interest to others. Details of this model can be obtained by writing the author of this paper.

References

Balderston, Frederick E. *Managing today's university*. San Francisco: Jossey-Bass, 1974.

Bean, Atherton. Fund raising and the trustee. *AGB Reports*, April 1973, *1*,6–12.

Bowen, Howard R. Finance and the aims of American higher education. In M. D. Orwig (Ed.), *Financing higher education*. Iowa City: Iowa: The American College Testing Program, 1971.

Boyer, Ernest L. A fresh look at the college trustee. *Educational Record*, Summer 1968, *49*,224–279.

Buchanan, James M., and Hartman, Robert W. Public finance and academic freedom: Consistency or contradictory? *AGB Reports*, January 1972, *14*,9–18.

Chambers, M. M. *Higher education: Who pays? Who gains?* Danville, Ill.: Interstate Printers & Publishers, Inc., 1968.

Green, Edith S. Issues in higher education. Proceedings of the 28th Annual Utah Conference on Higher Education, Utah State University, Logan, Utah, September 1971.

Hansen, W. Lee, and Weisbrod, Burton H. *Benefits, costs and finance of public higher education*. Chicago: Markham Publishing Company, 1969.

Harris, Seymour E. *A statistical portrait of higher education*. New York: McGraw-Hill, 1972.

Johns, R. L. The economics and financing of education. In Edgar L. Morphet and David L. Jesser (Eds.), *Designing education for the future*, No. 5. New York: Citation Press, 1968.

Johnson, Eldon L. Consortia in higher education. *Educational Record*, Fall 1967, *48*, 341–347.

Meeth, L. Richard. *Quality education for less money*. San Francisco: Jossey-Bass, 1974.

Milland, Richard M. State support for higher education. *AGB Reports*, May–June 1971, *13*,21–30.

Miner, Jerry. Financial support of education. In Edgar L. Morphet and David L. Jesser (Eds.), *Designing education for the future*, No. 5. New York: Citation Press, 1968.

Moore, R. S. *Consortia in American Higher Education 1965–66*. Washington, D.C.: U.S. Department of Health, Education and Welfare, 1968.

Morphet, Edgar L., and Jesser, David L. (Eds.), *Designing education for the future*, No. 5. New York: Citation Press, 1968.

Morse, John F. The federal government and higher education: General and specific concerns in the years ahead. *Educational Record*, Fall 1966, *47*,429–438.

Williams, Harry. *Planning for effective resource allocation in universities*. Washington, D.C.: American Council on Education, 1966.

Wood, Herbert H. Financial aspects of cooperation among institutions. In William W. Jellema (Ed.), *Efficient college management*. San Francisco: Jossey-Bass, 1972.

Special acknowledgement is made to M. David Hansen for providing this bibliography and other pertinent facts used in this paper.
A more comprehensive bibliography can be found in Franklin Patterson, *Colleges in consort*, San Francisco: Jossey-Bass, 1974.

Section Three

Manpower Needs and Career Opportunities

This section deals with issues relating to manpower needs in aging and career opportunities in the future. The questions addressed include: Who are we educating and training for what? What will the educated or trained person do? What about issues of licensing and credentialing? Without some ideas about what future needs will be, it is difficult to design current programs. At the same time, the increase in the number of programs educating and training people raises issues related to credentialing and licensing.

Professional Development and Credentialing in Gerontology

Donald L. Spence
University of Rhode Island

If we use as our standard the status of Fellow in the Gerontological Society then there are only three gerontologists in the State of Rhode Island. There are 150,000 people in the state who are 65 years or older. $1.8 million is spent annually on direct service programs. Approximately 7,900 are in institutions receiving total care. Overall some 7,500 people are employed in aging industries. Some are reasonably well trained for the job they are doing, and most have had some training in relation to their specific jobs, but few are educated with respect to the factual knowledge of aging, and therefore many perform their tasks using as a model the prejudices shared generally in our society concerning the aged, agism. Agism, as Butler (1975) calls it, perpetuates the myth of our elderly as: "as old as their years, as unproductive, as disengaged, as inflexible, as senile, or as living in a world of serenity." If people who are serving the elderly are aiding in the perpetuation of these myths and if most states have as few identified professionals per number of elderly as in Rhode Island, then the need for professional development in gerontology is without question.

Professional development, however, can take a number of forms. Up until last year the federal government, working with limited resources, tended to favor the short-term training of those people already in the field. Since this tended to place the control of training in the hands of those who needed it without specifying the training needed, it did not do a satisfactory job. Last year there was a shift in the direction of career training. With the federal government providing some direct support there has been a growing emergence of gerontology as a focus in many educational institutions throughout the country. Some indirect support for this development resulted from the money made available to Area Agencies on Aging for the encouragement of institutions of higher learning to offer gerontology courses at times and places convenient to those working in the field. Clearly the responsibility for professional development in aging is shifting in the direction of higher education. Given the limited training resources available in this situation of expanding programs, are we ready to accept the responsibility this entails both to the aged and to the agencies that serve the aged?

In any case, the present situation demands that we look carefully at those programs we intend to develop. What is our purpose in organizing and developing a gerontology program? Who are we planning to train? What resources do we have or do we need? What is our relationship to the other professions that provide service to the elderly? It is only when we have answers to these questions that we can know what a credential in gerontology will mean.

Purpose

In an address to a joint session at last year's Gerontological Society meeting, George Maddox made a distinction between education, training, and schooling which I have found extremely useful. By schooling he was referring to the organizational structure within which knowledge was transmitted. His distinction between education and training related to the content of that knowledge, where training meant the provision of specific skills to serve the elderly, and education meant attitudes and values based on a knowledge of the realities of aging rather than on supposition. Both forms of knowledge are necessary but in differing proportions depending on our objectives.

Certainly, there is some minimum level of education in aging required of any program which carries the label gerontology. But if all we provide is education in aging, then all we have produced is a new focus for the liberal arts. The issue is that between generalist and specialist and raises questions concerning the nature of specialties and whether these specialties should be focused on proactive or reactive problems of aging. The range of specialties is as broad as the total service spectrum within our society. The proactive/reactive focus is the traditional issue between prevention and treatment. The way you address these issues for your own program should help decide the proportions of education and training you need in your program.

Under ideal circumstances aging content would be part of traditional education with little need for exclusive gerontological focus. The psychologist or the nurse, the speech pathologist or the social worker, and the educator or the public administrator, in the regular course of their professional development, would learn the application of their art to an aging as well as to any population. Because this is not the case, we are confronted with the problems of: (1) how to get gerontological content into traditional professional training programs; or (2) what aspects of professional training need to be incorporated into gerontology. In the first instance we assume the professional training and provide education with respect to the application of that knowledge to the aged. In the second instance we assume the gerontological education and provide training in some professional skills as they relate to the aged. Our choice of program is dependent on both the student to whom it is directed and the available resources.

Students

The traditional student offers the greatest potential in terms of the widest possible range of gerontological offerings. Even if a gerontology program offers no marketable skills it can still serve its students by providing education for living throughout life, freed of the prejudices which mar the lives of so many of today's older citizens. In essence, such a program could complement the usual psychology and sociology undergraduate programs that prepare the student for living, but not for making a living. Since many traditional students are expecting to find work upon completion of their undergraduate education the combination of gerontology with the skills of such disciplines as education, nursing, home economics, journalism, dental hygiene, medical technology, etc., can be extremely appealing.

At the other extreme is the most difficult student for whom to develop a program, the employed practitioner. Since he/she theoretically has the skills for his/her job, education in aging is what is needed, but not necessarily what is wanted. They are usually busy people who look upon course work as a means of developing skills that can either make their job easier or earn them more money, i.e., training. Education, on the other hand, takes time and since they are presently involved with the aged it is difficult to convince them that they must spend hours learning about people they already presume to know.

Experience with the elderly is not necessarily a good teacher. It has been shown that the exposure of medical students to older patients tends to reinforce prejudices. They see the aged in a dependent sick role from which they seem to generalize (Spence, Feigenbaum, Fitzgerald, and Roth, 1968). I continually ask myself how many service workers with the elderly are similarly affected? The trained person may have the skills to deal effectively with his/her client. But only the educated person really understands why the client is there and how under other circumstances the situation might be reversed.

A final category of student any program must consider is the older student who is beginning another career. This is particularly important in relation to professional development within gerontology. The gerontology industries are primarily service industries which are directed toward a population with limited financial resources. In order to maximize those services, the aged themselves must be encouraged to function to the optimum of their capabilities and interests. If we do not encourage this, then we are the worst kind of parasite, benefiting from the services we provide the elderly while our actions deprive the elderly of altering their situation so as not to need our services.

Gerontology should have as its professional maxim, "Do for the elderly only that which they cannot do for themselves, continually trying to work yourself out of a job." There is still plenty to be done. The elderly themselves are among those who practice agism most frequently. Through the education and training of older students to provide services for their peers, we maintain the resources within the population needing the service.

Resources

The elderly are seen as a principal resource in the development of gerontology programs. Supposedly, the student as a service provider gains experience in his/her direct involvement with this client group. As Eric Pfeiffer (1977) has indicated, however, unsupervised experience with the elderly does not improve the quality of services delivered. This points to one of the thorniest issues in gerontology today, i.e., who has the qualifications to provide professional development in gerontology?

Professional development involves a process of socialization. To be educated in the subject areas of gerontology by someone who has not himself/ herself been previously socialized is like taking a course in union organizing from a management personnel officer. It takes more than knowledge of a subject to socialize others; it takes a commitment to the application of this knowledge in specified ways. If we are going to use the field as our classroom then we had better make sure that we have the supervisory personnel to train the student as he/she works. Whether field supervisor or classroom teacher, the problem is how to develop this trained personnel.

One does not become a gerontologist by a quickie exposure to its subject matter in a summer institute. Summer institutes are excellent ways of learning about new developments, curricula, or other resources in the field, but they cannot substitute for formal professionalization in gerontology. Formal professionalization takes time. A program can either hire the trained professional or provide the time for existing staff to become re-educated in gerontology. In either case it involves an institutional commitment.

Administrative support is a key to the success of professional development. The commitment has to begin at the top if we are to build teaching, curricular, and library resources along with meeting our manpower needs. It is one thing to direct unused resources to gerontology regardless of their appropriateness; it is quite another to invest in the development of quality programming. Since gerontology is an interdisciplinary field the task need not be overwhelming.

Returning to our earlier distinction of either adding gerontology to professional training or professional skills to gerontological training, the choice should be evident. A limited number of resources can provide gerontological input into the training of any number of professionals, but to develop a degree program in gerontology requires substantial resources. It is understandable for the University of Southern California to develop a degree program in gerontology. They have the resources to justify such a degree. Without those resources, a gerontology degree usually means an aging focus to social psychological training. If we are ever going to certify professionals in gerontology, then the certification should mean what it says. I believe that an honest statement of our *capabilities* and *limitations* is the only position that will promote the kind of interprofessional relationships needed for the effective development and credentialing of professionals in gerontology.

References

Butler, R. N. *Why survive? Being old in America*. New York: Harper & Row, 1975.
Pfeiffer, E. Legislative action—the needed first step in strengthening faculty and curricula. *Geriatrics*, January 1977, *32*(1), 105–106.
Spence, D. L., Feigenbaum, E. M., Fitzgerald, F., and Roth, J. Medical student attitudes toward the geriatric patient. *Journal of the American Geriatrics Society*, 1968, *16*,976–983.

New Career Opportunities in Gerontology for the 1980s: A Crystal Ball

Roger Hiemstra
Iowa State University

I would like to present a few introductory remarks in the area of new career opportunities in gerontology. My suggestions are intended primarily as stimulators for your initial thinking on new career opportunities in gerontology.

Societal interest in, and pressures for, increased attention to gerontology are mounting. This increasing interest can be documented in many ways. Increasing enrollments by older adults in all forms of learning, the fact that older persons are making their needs known, and the growing number of professionals becoming involved with gerontology programs are some of the areas where figures can be obtained.

There are other kinds of forces creating pressures that affect the older person. The *Future Shock* theme of rapid change and several hypothesized adjustment problems, the spiraling inflation and its negative impact on fixed incomes, and the changing societal values or life styles as evidenced by the "back to earth" movement that tend to create greater intergenerational conflicts are only some of those that could be mentioned. You may be able to list several other forces or changes.

What does this all mean for career opportunities in gerontology for the 1980s?

I would like to list a few changes I see taking place that have implications for new career possibilities. You will note that I'm looking at career opportunities fairly narrowly, i.e., through adult education eyes or the training of educators to work with the older adult. Some points are very service oriented, some are training oriented, some are research oriented in implication, and others are new, different, evolving, or speculative in nature.

1. The counseling area—adult educators are just beginning to obtain the skills necessary to counsel with adult students. I'm convinced that this will spill over, if it hasn't already, into the older adult arena.
2. Community colleges and the older adult—there are already several good examples of community colleges operating successful programs for older adult learners. I think that such models will facilitate a rapid expansion of like programs across the country.
3. The self-directed learner—there is considerable evidence that much of the adult learning that takes place is not carried out within a classroom setting. This has been found to be true for older as well as younger adults. Subsequently, the whole nontraditional education movement is about to discover the older adult.
4. Volunteer training—the RSVP and other similar programs are beginning to involve thousands of older persons throughout the country. As this movement grows, individuals who can carry out the needed training and coordinate the volunteer activities will be increasingly needed.
5. Lifelong learning legislation—the recent passage of lifelong learning legislation as a part of the Higher Education Act has unknown implications for the fields of adult education and gerontology. The intensive discussion and lobbying now taking place on that legislation indicates the intense interest and the potentially huge impact on the American society. I have no doubt that related career opportunities in gerontology will exist and increase in a very short period of time.
6. Consumer education interest—the high interest in consumer education, consumer protection, etc., is beginning to include more attention on the older adult consumer. Subsequently, people who can present consumer education programs to the older person, who can carry out research in this area, and who can speak as a voice for the older person on consumer topics will be needed.
7. Understanding of one's self—I believe that there will be an increasing need for and interest in an understanding of self and what is happening during the aging process by older persons. Thus, there should be career potential in the area of teaching older adults about what is happening to them.

There are several other ideas I did not mention that were nicely highlighted in the Fall, 1976, issue of *Occupational Outlook Quarterly*. This was a special issue on "Working with Older People." A few other references of considerable interest are available from the author upon request.

One final thought: It seems to me that we, those in the field of gerontology or those interested in the field, need to take a more careful look at occupation opportunities and how we prepare people to work in the various occupations. This means examining ourselves not only in terms of the professional versus the academic preparation paradigm suggested by Dave Peterson, but also in terms of different areas or classifications of preparation, such as service, training, or research oriented areas. Once we do this, different higher education institutions can begin to develop preparation programs with some direction.

References

Toffler, Alvin. *Future shock*. New York: Random House, 1970.
U.S. Department of Labor, Bureau of Labor Statistics. *Occupational Quarterly*, Fall 1976.

Manpower Needs in Aging:
A Look at the Marketplace

Richard Schloss
Administration on Aging

One of the phenomena that has never ceased to amaze me during the time that I have worked in aging is that so many of the major concerns and issues persist, and that progress towards their resolution is slow in coming. This was brought home to me again recently when I had occasion to refer to some of the material for the 1971 White House Conference on Aging. The Background and Issues paper prepared on training reads, in some respects, as if it had been written only yesterday.

That survey of the manpower situation in 1970 revealed the existence of a large number of persons working in aging, at different levels of responsibility, that called for varying degrees of broad interaction with older persons. A broad survey of the field today would yield comparable findings. These characteristics represent the challenge and dilemma confronting all of us who are concerned with training in aging, for many of the issues reflected by the 1971 White House Conference remain with us: Given a limitation on available public resources, what are the priorities for who should be trained and at what level; what are the respective roles to be assumed by government as well as the educational and professional community in ensuring that an adequate number of qualified persons are working in the field of aging; and, what are the organizational configurations most effective to accomplish these tasks? The difficulties associated with reaching decisions concerning training priorities and appropriate approaches are shared by officials of public funding agencies, educational institutions, and professional organizations. As the competition for available resources increases, a critical factor which increasingly we all will be obligated to consider in our requests and justifications for aging training support is the extent to which that request addresses the current and projected need for personnel in the field of aging. Faculty and deans alike are becoming increasingly aware that an educational institution which is considering the introduction or development of gerontology capability must assess the marketplace implications of such an action. The relative merits of an institutional investment of current and future resources to training in gerontology are being measured against the commitment of those same resources to support other program areas. Need, as reflected by the marketplace, can tip the balance of the decision-making process.

Data Collection and Analysis

Having said that, let me add that when I look into the crystal ball to project the manpower needs in aging for the 1980s, it looks very cloudy. I'm referring to a cloudiness of vision, rather than to a negative prediction of employment opportunities in the field. The fact is that there are relatively little data available on which to make quantitative projections for the various occupations and industries that can and do serve the needs of older persons.

Though there are many techniques and approaches available for obtaining data and assessing manpower needs, a problem for the aging field exists in the definition and classification of the aging relatedness of the various occupations that comprise the aging manpower pool. This is the principal reason for the lack of data available for publication. Some occupations concern themselves exclusively or primarily with aging or older persons. Those occupations associated with the nursing home industry, or homemaker-home health aides, or persons working in aging network agencies, fall into this category. On the other hand, a great many persons work with or on behalf of older persons as part of their work with the population at large. It is this characteristic of the aging manpower pool that makes data collection and analysis difficult and prohibitively expensive, for it is difficult to separate the aging-exclusive personnel requirements of an occupation from those related to serving all people. Social workers, public administrators, health workers, architects, lawyers, and so forth, all can and do serve the elderly. Employment projections have been developed for these and many other occupations on an as it is currently collected and analyzed.

There have been a few efforts during the past 10 years to fill this need for manpower information in aging. A major study authorized by the Congress was undertaken in 1968 for the Administration on Aging entitled *The Demand for Personnel and Training in the Field of Aging*. It highlighted major shortages of trained and specialized personnel in programs serving the aging, including professional positions in federal and state agencies on aging, and management and other personnel for retirement housing, recreation, and long-term care facilities.

The 1973 Amendments to the Older Americans Act broadened the Title IV-A manpower analysis authority of the Administration on Aging. Since the 1973 amendments the AoA, through the Division of Manpower Resources, has initiated a number of activities that are directed to making information available to assist those who must make decisions affecting training and manpower development in aging. Materials, in the form of reports and analyses, have been and are being developed. Public hearings and conferences have been held and publication of the proceedings is in process. The outcome of these efforts, it is hoped, will be more and better data and other information that is relevant to the needs of administrators, researchers, educators, and the public.

The Bureau of Labor Statistics, of the Department of Labor, has assisted AoA in carrying many of these manpower related activities. Two analyses of aging-specific occupations have been completed by BLS. One, *Manpower Needs in the Field of Aging: The Nursing Home Industry* was published and distributed by AoA as the initial item in a new publication series, "AoA Occasional Papers in Gerontology." Because of limitations in the AoA printing budget, the word *occasional* took on special significance—there hasn't been another publication in the series since last year. However, the study entitled *Human Resource Issues in the Field of Aging: Homemaker-Home Health Aide Services* is now at the printers and should be available as Occasional Paper Number 2 within six weeks.[1] Both of these studies analyzed basic employment data and other research that already was available.

Factors Affecting Employment

Projections of the number of persons needed in the field, or the number to be trained, are only a part of the manpower assessment picture. Adding to the data collection and classification problems for aging-related occupations are several interrelated manifestations of the employment market that complicate the overall analysis of aging manpower needs. The causes and effects of turnover, barriers to entry and advancement in the field, the problems associated with attracting persons to aging, and training and education needs are other components of the manpower mosaic that require understanding and analysis.

In order to gain a sense of the importance of these marketplace characteristics, AoA initiated several forums of discussion designed to elicit a broad variety of opinion and reaction. During the spring of 1976 the Commissioner on Aging held three public hearings around the country to discuss the manpower needs in social services for the elderly. Testimony was presented on behalf of state and area agencies on aging, consumers, educators, professional associations, service providers, and others. A summary of the hearings will be published shortly. In addition, AoA sponsored the conduct of two small conferences of practitioners and educators to examine the question of the adequacy of trained persons to work with the elderly; one addressed the manpower needs related to state and area agencies on aging, and the other to the needs in the social work profession. The intent of these conferences was the identification of issues, trends, information gaps, potential areas for research, and demonstration related to the workings of the employment market and the manpower needs. Conference reports will be completed later this year.

A discussion follows of four factors which characterize the workings of the aging employment market as revealed by the conferences, hearings, and related research: recruitment, turnover, barriers to utilization, and training.[2]

1. Recruitment. Many of the positions in the field of aging, both service-related occupations as well as administrative, are relatively lower paying and have fewer benefits than do comparable positions in other fields. Thus, while there may be qualified persons to fill available positions, they may choose comparable jobs in other fields. For instance, examples have been cited where area agencies have had difficulty in recruiting social workers because of the higher salary and prestige offered by a State Department of Welfare or a State Department of Mental Health. This, combined with concerns for acceptable working conditions and limited prospects for advancement, can create serious barriers to recruiting people into the field.

Though low pay and limited opportunities for advancement are negative factors to attracting people to the field, recruiting applicants with adequate qualifications does not appear to be a problem. The supply of persons available for direct service jobs in aging is generally adequate, and in urban areas may be abundant. Professional and administrative jobs in state and area agencies on aging and service-providing organizations also attract more highly qualified persons than are needed. Many of the applicants are recent college graduates, with unrelated degrees, who nevertheless qualify according to position classification standards. In-service training was seen as one realistic means of meeting the gerontology and other knowledge gaps of these otherwise qualified persons.

Applicants are attracted by (1) a desire to help the elderly, (2) the status of "acceptability" that the field is earning, (3) the security resulting from the pending growth of services to the elderly, and (4) the newness of the field that allows for more creativity than in established social service areas. Limits on earnings and mobility within the field may lead eventually to transfer out of the field.

2. Turnover. While a certain amount of turnover can be expected in any field due to workers changing jobs, moving, retiring, or leaving the work force for other reasons, when it is excessive it may be symptomatic of a manpower problem. In all of the studies conducted for AoA by the Labor Department, turnover was identified as being a frequently occurring phenomenon. In both the nursing home and homemaker-home health aide studies, projected annual openings resulting from persons who transfer out of the occupation are far greater than those resulting from growth. Reasons for transfer out included dislike of the work, low wages or benefits, inability to cope with depressed or difficult clients. Turnover is prevalent also in many state and area aging agencies. The principle reason cited was the lack of career ladders, which results in the need for employees to agency-hop in order to get ahead. Because of this deficiency, most employees attain their maximum growth potential in aging and transfer out of the field.

Turnover has been viewed by many as a plus to the field of aging because it keeps new fresh talent coming in, and it results in a diffusion of expertise whereby new agencies and organizations that previously were not sensitive to the needs of older persons now have resident experience and expertise in aging. However, when viewed from the perspective of an individual agency the negative aspects of turnover can be quite detrimental. Continuity of programs is difficult to achieve since it is harder to maintain a consistent quality and volume of service when workers continually leave and must be replaced. Secondly, when an agency is temporarily shorthanded it places an additional burden on the remaining workers until a replacement is found. Thirdly, a considerable amount of administrative time is spent recruiting and hiring new employees rather than being devoted to other tasks. And finally, training funds and staff time, both of which are always in short supply, are devoted to maintaining a given level of staff competence rather than improving it.

The lack of career ladders was cited by many as a particularly acute problem relating to both recruitment and turnover. In the administrative fields, particularly in state and area agencies, it was noted that many of these agencies are small and offer extremely limited opportunities for growth and advancement. Because of the low salaries, many recent graduates take these jobs as entry level positions that provide needed experience in order to qualify themselves for higher paying positions in other fields. The growth of the aging network as a network may offer some increased career opportunities. However, the impression among those with whom we discussed this issue was that movement among administrative persons and program specialists in social service programs was more likely to occur laterally, from program to program at the same administrative level and the same geographic area, rather than vertically, from one administrative level to another within the same program area. An agency area person, it was thought, is more likely to move to an employment or housing program in the same community, than he is to move to a state agency or aging position within the same or another state.

3. Barriers to Utilization. A variety of regulations and administrative procedures exacerbate the foregoing problems by creating barriers to effective utilization of adequately trained persons. This should be an area of particular concern to those in institutions of higher education. Students graduating with particular knowledge and skills in gerontology are confronted with the problems of qualifying for positions which are vacant.

The most frequently cited problem is related to civil service requirements and restrictions which govern not only qualification criteria for positions, but the salary and benefit levels as well. As the aging network has grown and developed, increasingly these agencies are subject to state, county, or local civil service requirements. The problem for those of us concerned with aging is that the qualifications for many aging agency staff positions are not specific to the field of aging, and that personnel systems have been slow to recognize the desirability of gerontology training for many aging jobs. The net result of this is that graduates from aging training programs may be handicapped in their competition for jobs. Persons without education or experience in the field of aging often come out among those most highly qualified on the list of eligibles because the evaluation criteria do not reflect the need for a gerontology background. Selection generally comes from the top of the list and the individual with a specialized aging background is often denied the position.

Another manifestation of that same situation is that the position is "underclassified" in that qualifications are not of a sufficient professional nature to command a salary level that would attract persons with aging training and experience.

Finally, for a variety of reasons including the current unemployment situation, some state civil service systems will only consider seriously applications from residents of that state. In such cases, of course, the recent graduate who perceives that he or she is mobile and willing to relocate is actually much more limited in the options available. Such a situation is not unique to the aging field but can and does affect some who are seeking employment in aging.

4. Training. Two training related themes emerged from the conferences and public hearings: the need for in-service training, and concern over the job market for college graduates with preservice training in gerontology.

Many newly hired paraprofessionals and professionals require training to build job skills and to correct misconceptions about aging and the aged. Often professionals, administrators, and paraprofessionals who are currently working in social service programs have little knowledge of the aging process or of the skills needed to work with the elderly. It was felt that, as a consequence, the planning and delivery of services to older persons suffer. The linking of in-service programs into academically based or affiliated programs aimed at giving a person a well-rounded background in aging emerged as a means of improving an employee's performance and, at the same time, increasing both the worker's commitment to aging and chances of mobility within the field.

Some people felt that job related training, particularly for network agency personnel, was best provided by those working in the network. As a consequence of their familiarity with the needs, problems, and perspective of network employees, it was felt that training content would be more compatible and relevant to worker needs than it would be if the training was designed, developed, and delivered by institutionally based academicians or staff from management and other consulting firms. This appears to be an area where better understanding will be gained through discussions and cooperative efforts between the communities of education and practice.

There was some feeling that graduates of baccalaureate and graduate multidisciplinary programs were having difficulty finding jobs in aging. The combination of the barriers to the effective use of qualified persons cited earlier, and the apparent availability of highly qualified persons to accept vacant jobs, may well account for this situation. No evidence was presented, but it is a question of concern to all of us, and one which AoA now is looking into as part of an evaluation of the career training program. At the same time, increased gerontology training within professional disciplines such as social work, law, and the various health professions was encouraged.

Manpower Trends

I would like to point up several tentative observations that have emerged from these forums concerning the manpower trends in the field and to conclude with some thoughts on the response of educational institutions to the manpower needs we have discussed.

The following items characterize the emerging trends:

◆ An increase in the number of professional and paraprofessional service delivery jobs is likely, with the corresponding need to train persons to assume supervisory roles.

◆ Employment requirements of state and area agencies on aging are limited and the rapid employment growth of the past several years will not continue. Employment in state agencies is determined mainly by federal (Older Americans Act) and state level funding whose limits will restrict growth. Area agencies, with additional potential sources of support such as local funds, CETA, VISTA, Title IX, and revenue sharing, may grow somewhat more, but the long-range prospect remains for limited growth.

◆ As agencies mature, the nature of the jobs change, often requiring more sophisticated knowledge and abilities. Future requirements may call for agencies with fewer persons giving basic technical assistance for service development, and increased requirements for persons trained in planning social service systems and in public finance.

◆ As older persons gain financial and physical access to an increased range of social and health services, there will be an increased demand for these services, with a corresponding need for increased gerontology training within the established disciplines and professions, such as law, medicine, nursing, public administration, and social work.

◆ Social services needs to minority elderly are not being met now, and the situation will continue to exacerbate unless there is a significant increase in the number of minority professionals available for training, planning, administrative and direct service jobs in aging. Similarly, a need exists for increased numbers of researchers and educators who are representative of minority groups.

Conclusion

In the light of this discussion of manpower needs, three areas suggest themselves for consideration.

First, consideration of the marketplace should become an increasingly significant factor in the determination of training policy and priorities. The education community should continue its own discussions of policy directions in the light of the marketplace, and should work with the public agencies and others to develop significant manpower data needs and recommend steps to fill the data gaps. More attention, too, should be given to analysis and interpretation of existing manpower data on aging. In general, I feel the questions of marketplace needs, and the workings of the marketplace, are an appropriate item that should be considered by educators and trainers in the classroom as well as in planning agenda for professional meetings.

For its part the Administration on Aging is moving toward filling some of the information and data gaps during this current year. As I mentioned earlier, as part of the evaluation of the career training program, we will be looking at the employment histories of graduates of the gerontology training programs supported by AoA. Secondly, we are exploring the feasibility of adding gerontology related employment questions into the general employment surveys of a number of federal agencies. If this proves workable, the data base for the aging specific portion of general population oriented occupations will be greatly increased. Thirdly, the nursing home industry study will be updated this year as more current information has been collected. Finally, a second special issue of the *Occupational Outlook Quarterly*, comparable to the one you have received in your packets, will be developed this year. While the current issue focuses on service occupations, the new one will deal with the professions.

Second, increased attention should be given to marketplace considerations by those planning to develop a gerontology program, as well as for those with one already established. One consideration in assessing the costs and benefits of the type and resource commitment necessary to build a program should be the expected employment success of the graduates. Questions of level of training, nature of the credential offered, the administrative structure of the program within the institution—these and many more issues must be addressed in determining how best to design a program that will provide the knowledge and skills graduates will take with them into the marketplace. In addition, given the diversity of training needs, an institution should consider what role is appropriate and desirable for it to play in meeting those needs; what particular marketplace need is it meeting, is it a unique role, or is it one being shared with few or many other institutions serving the same market? Gerontology program planning and development should include such considerations.

Third, the growing interdependency of interests between the educational community and the agencies of the aging network suggests the advantages of a considered effort to work more closely on an ongoing basis. Such a cooperative effort has the potential benefit of making the educational resources increasingly relevant and responsive to the changing marketplace needs of both agency practitioners and preservice students. It could also afford increased employment and practicum opportunities for students. Equally important, gerontology expertise remains a relatively scarce commodity which, when available, should be maximized to its fullest. Cooperation between educational institutions and network agencies can result in better planning and coordination of the gerontology training resources available in the state or region. This would ensure that, to the extent that resources allow, priority needs are met for undergraduate, graduate, professional, and in-service training in aging.

Meeting the manpower needs in the field of aging is the collective concern of all of us who are interested in education and training. It is important that vocationally oriented training programs, such as gerontology, reflect in their planning and in their conduct an understanding of the workings and demands of the marketplace into which their graduates will pass. Discussion of manpower needs, such as this one today, have with more frequency become part of the formal agenda of meetings of educators and trainers. This is a positive step that will add a significant dimension to the ongoing discussion of priority setting, resource allocation, and the development of training programs responsive to current and future manpower needs.

References

Birren, James E., et al. *Training: Background and issues.* White House Conference on Aging. Washington, D.C., 1971. Out of print.

U.S. Department of Health, Education, and Welfare, Administration on Aging. *The demand for personnel and training in the field of aging* (AoA Publication No. 270). Washington, D.C., July 1969. Out of print.

U.S. Department of Health, Education, and Welfare, Administration on

Aging. *Manpower needs in the field of aging: The nursing home industry* [AoA Occasional Papers in Gerontology, No. 1, DHEW Publications No. (OHD) 76-20082]. Washington, D.C., 1976. Out of print.

U.S. Department of Health, Education, and Welfare, Administration on Aging. *Human resource issues in the field of aging: Homemaker-home health aide services* (AoA Occasional Papers in Gerontology, No. 2). Washington, D.C., in press.

Notes

1. Editors' note: At the time this book went to press, this study and the reports of other studies mentioned in this article were still not available.

2. The following discussion draws heavily on draft material developed by staff of the Bureau of Labor Statistics as part of their preparation and summarization of the manpower hearings and the two conferences.

New Career Opportunities in Gerontology in the 1980s: Research and Teaching

Erdman Palmore
Duke University

More Careers

Perhaps the most important thing to recognize about new careers in gerontology is that in the 1980s there will probably be more of them than ever before. All signs point in the direction of continued growth in most areas of gerontology.

Those of you who are new to the field may not know about the remarkable growth in gerontology. The statistics are dramatic. A generation ago there were hardly any gerontologists identified as such. Now there are about 4,000 professional members of the Gerontological Society. A generation ago there were almost no courses offered in gerontology. Now there are literally thousands of such courses in over 800 colleges and in more than 400 community and junior colleges across the United States. A generation ago there were no centers for the study of aging. Now there are about two dozen major centers primarily devoted to research and teaching in gerontology. The 1976 *National Directory of Programs in Gerontology* prepared by AGHE lists 1,275 programs, and this does not include some that were overlooked and the many programs that have started since the Directory came out. A generation ago there were no journals in gerontology; now there are at least six professional journals and a couple of dozen popular journals and "newsletters" in aging.

Even the federal government has finally established a National Institute on Aging. Thus, the past dramatic growth is well documented.

The big question, of course, is "Will this growth continue in the 1980s?" I think the answer is probably "Yes," unless there is nuclear war or some other major disaster. The number of people over age 65 will continue to grow at a faster rate than the rest of the population, and the numbers over age 75 who need more programs and services will continue to grow at an even faster rate. Perhaps more importantly, more and more older and *younger people* recognize the problems and neglected potential of the aged, and they are demanding more and more adequate programs for the aged. Responding to this demand, the federal government has continued to increase its programs for the aged and for research and teaching in gerontology (for which the Association for Gerontology in Higher Education deserves much credit). I can see no signs that these trends would be reversed in the 1980s. If anything, the Carter Administration (with our own Juanita Kreps on the cabinet) promises to be *more* favorable to aging and gerontology than the past administrations.

Therefore, I think it is safe to predict for the 1980s a continuing increase in the number and variety of new careers in gerontology.

Evaluation Research

The other authors of this section will talk about new careers in administration and service. I want to discuss new careers—or changing emphases—in research and teaching centers. One growing emphasis is on evaluation research. Too often in the past big and little programs and projects and "demonstrations" have been set up, and collapsed as soon as the grants ran out, partly because there was little or no evaluation built into the project to determine whether the project did any good at all, much less whether it actually achieved its stated goals, or whether its benefit/cost ratio was high or low. Thus, they were unable to prove that the project was worth continued funding from any source. All they demonstrated was that people could be organized to spend whatever funds were available in an attempt to deliver some kind of "service" or another. More and more public and private agencies are recognizing that this is not good enough, and are requiring that each project devote some part of its budget to an objective evaluation of its effectiveness and benefits, relative to its costs. Evaluation research is challenging at best, usually difficult, and often frustrating for a number of reasons, such as the difficulty of accurately measuring benefits, outcomes, or improvements in the quality of life, the difficulty of setting up appropriate control groups, the difficulty of controlling for other factors that may be involved, and so forth. But good, important research is always difficult and often frustrating. In any case, I believe this growing recognition of the need for good evaluation of the thousands of projects being undertaken in gerontology will lead to more new careers specializing in evaluation research.

Interdisciplinary Careers

A second growing emphasis is on interdisciplinary research and teaching. Too often in the past, specialists in each of the disciplines have either ignored the contributions of specialists from other disciplines or they have attacked each other's domains in petty attempts to enlarge their own domains. I think there is growing recognition that gerontology is by nature an interdisciplinary venture, which cuts across most of the traditional disciplines, and that attempts to ignore any of these disciplines or to quarrel over boundary lines only weakens gerontology. Fortunately, the Duke Center for the Study of Aging was founded on an interdisciplinary principle and I can report that we work hard trying to work together, regardless of our specialty training, and we are convinced that this effort is worthwhile. I still believe that the best researchers start out with a thorough training in one of the traditional disciplines before specializing in gerontology, but there are those who disagree, and I recognize that this may be less important in teaching. In any case, I think these interdisciplinary trends will continue so that there will be more opportunities in the 1980s for interdisciplinary careers and cooperation.

Intercultural Gerontology

A third growing emphasis in gerontology is international and interethnic research and teaching. There are now three international organizations in gerontology: the International Association of Gerontology, the International Center of Social Gerontology, and the International Federation on Aging. In the last 10 years numerous articles and several books have appeared on international gerontology. I am now editing an *International Handbook on Aging* which we hope will be ready for the 1978 International Congress of Gerontology in Tokyo. It will include chapters on gerontology in some thirty different countries. For several years the United States Gerontological Society has had a subcommittee on International Research. This year the committee has been broadened to include interethnic research as well, and has been renamed the subcommittee on Intercultural Research. We are trying to stimulate, organize, and disseminate more research and teaching in this broad area on the basic principle that in order to become a truly comprehensive and universal science, gerontology must study and teach about aging around the world and in many different ethnic and racial groups. Too often in the past gerontologists have had a rather parochial view, limited mainly to white Anglo-Saxon Americans. I think the 1980s will bring more and more interest, research, and teaching in a broader intercultural view of gerontology.

Less Dependency

The fourth, and final, trend that I believe will affect careers in gerontology is the trend toward better health and higher socioeconomic status among the aged. Many gerontologists have known for some time that the average health, education, previous occupation, and income of the aged have been improving slowly. But until recently there has been some question as to whether the aged were keeping up with the improvements in these areas among the rest of the population. Now it appears that not only are the aged keeping up, but [they] are actually reducing the gaps between them and younger people in terms of health, education, lifetime occupations, and income (Palmore, 1976). The reasons for these shifts toward better health and socioeconomic status are complex, and appear to involve slowing rates of social change and the many new and improved programs for the aged such as Medicare, the Supplementary Security Income programs, better pension and social security benefits, etc. But the main point for future careers in gerontology is that the future aged population is becoming less dependent, less in need of welfare type services, and more independent, more able to *buy* the services they want.

Another trend that points in the same direction is the trend toward early retirement, so that more and more people have the opportunity and are choosing to retire on comfortable incomes at younger ages. Already the majority of new social security beneficiaries are choosing to retire *before* age 65. It is becoming common for people in certain occupations to "retire" in their late 50's or earlier, even though they may go back to work part-time, or even full-time, in a "second career." This growing group of "young-old" as they have been called, or the "early-retired" as I would call them, are even healthier, have more income, education, and higher previous occupations than other older persons.

Perhaps you can already see the implications for gerontologists. These trends should result in less of the welfare-worker and pauper roles, and more of the counselor and client roles; less of the healthy middle-class professor studying the infirm and poverty-stricken aged, and more studies of the leisure and work patterns of the comfortable and active majority of aged—many of whom may have incomes higher than the professor's. It may mean less rescuing those few aged who have been defeated by the crises of retirement or widowhood, and more preretirement counseling so that more retirees will better adjust to the problems of retirement and aging. Just as many health professionals are shifting from treating the already sick to preventive medicine among the well, perhaps many gerontologists can shift from rescue operations to planning and prevention services.

As a specific example of the kind of career I would expect to grow because of these trends, consider retirement planning and counseling. Here is a service which has repeatedly shown beneficial results, and researchers at Duke, Drake, Southern California, Chicago, and elsewhere are developing more and better models for various types of situations. Yet surveys indicate that only about one in 10 corporations offer any kind of comprehensive retirement information and counseling service to their employees. Think of the new careers that would open up if even half the corporations started offering such services!

Summary

My crystal ball tells me that the 1980s will bring more and more varied careers in gerontology, and that areas of unusual opportunity will develop in evaluation research, interdisciplinary research and teaching, international and interethnic gerontology, and such counselor-client careers as retirement planning and counseling. My crystal ball does show some threatening clouds around the edges that indicate the possibility of various disasters such as nuclear war, world-wide depression, or exhaustion of energy resources; but the dominant picture seems to be one of blue skies and mild weather.

References

Palmore, E. The future status of the aged. *Gerontologist*, 1976, *16*(4),297–302.

Sprouse, B. *National directory of programs in gerontology*. Madison: University of Wisconsin Press, 1976.

Section Four

Special Service Aspects
of College and University Programs

Most colleges and universities have explicitly defined public service functions. Schools with gerontology courses or programs must meet the obligations of their schools' mission statements. Additionally, each program often has an implicit service ideology unique to that particular program. These ideologies may emphasize providing short-term training activities for practitioners, programs for older adults, consulting services, or various forms of research activities. The following papers deal with some of the issues relating to schools' service functions and crystallize some of the concerns people have regarding the relationships between school and community.

Issues of Services

Ira F. Ehrlich
Southern Illinois University

In discussing the relationship of higher education to the issues of services, I'd like to begin by making two assumptions:

1. Higher education (HE) cannot be everything to everybody. This
means that institutions or programs of HE do not have the resources to
provide all the necessary gerontological training/education and research for a
total community. Therefore, HE must be able to make choices of what it can
and will offer to a community.

2. Every HE program/institution has uniqueness: strengths which
should guide its choice of what it does offer on a qualitative basis.

To assist our focusing on the issues I am going to state six principles.
These are:

1. The *major* role of an institution dedicated or sanctioned to offer HE is
education. However, educational aspects may include service components.
Thus, the educational role per se is not mutually exclusive.

2. A university and/or other institution of HE has both the sanction and
the resources to develop and test knowledge particularly in new content areas.
This role as it relates to service may be implemented through an emphasis on
applied research and demonstration. In this role there is need for cooperation

between the university and the community formal service system in order that the university's demonstration can become integrated into the community service system when the university research role is terminated. Such an example of knowledge development by and for new content areas through applied research and demonstration was the development of the elderly single room occupants (SRO's) study, service, and policy oriented program developed at the Institute of Applied Gerontology (IAG).[1]

3. HE in gerontology has the unique opportunity to develop an institution-wide policy of multi- and/or interdisciplinary education as the sanctioned approach to gerontology programs. Such a universal policy, e.g., in a university desirous to create/develop gerontology programs, would tend to have an immediate (and expected positive) effect as a model for service development.

4. If an institution of HE is to establish standards for gerontological education/training then such concerns include who is to be trained and what are the best (at times innovative) approaches to accomplish this task. This seems to suggest that repeated "one-day" programs and rating on training "low level people" who tend to have short job tenure may be a questionable priority for the regular utilization of today's generally limited resources of HE.

5. In this increasingly complex and specialized world in which HE gerontology needs to function there is need for "field and/or applied" experience for faculty/staff responsible for varied gerontological programs. Faculty thus need to use themselves in some "doing" relation in service (including politics). This "special assignment" sabbatical or more frequent "applied/field" approach will tend to assist classroom academic faculty to be more in tune with services and models needed for services.

6. HE in gerontology has the sanction and the resources to upgrade education for a variety of target populations. Two prime examples of this potential educational service need are:

a. Intensive education for current professionals in the field; and

b. The elderly as consumers and/or developers of higher education.

Note

1. Further information about this research/educational service model can be obtained from the author.

Academic Gerontology and the Community: Love-Hate Relationships

Lillian Troll
Rutgers University
Jody Olsen
University of Maryland

Community Perspectives

It is important that those developing new knowledge in and training people for work in gerontology work closely with those who design, plan, and deliver services to older people. Only through mutual respect and understanding can each carry out his task and use resources more fully. Therefore, before an educational institution can share with the community training and research resources or draw services from it, it must understand how the community of service givers sees itself and the educational institution. In the following discussion we examine some of these ways.

First, community workers have a strong working knowledge about those they serve, and are proud of this knowledge. Working daily with a group of people builds an "instinctive" sense about the people's needs, how they act, what changes they are seeking, and how others can be helpful to them. How can anyone else acquire this same knowledge? In dealing with other professionals, service givers want to be recognized for the knowledge developed through their work. When practitioners are given recognition for this knowledge, it is easier for them to then accept further information and training that might be available.

Second, those working in the community are looking for support for what they do. Many feel that their jobs are difficult and that recognition of these difficult tasks is important to their ability to continue. This recognition is particularly important for people providing direct services. There are tremendous emotional commitments made in direct service which can be emotionally wearing without proper recognition of their accomplishments. Training programs and other consultative work should build in a component that recognizes this need for support.

Third, many community professionals feel that they have either had too much training or the wrong kind of training. Because their time is important, they feel it crucial that the training and technical assistance they are involved in be what they perceive as meaningful. For this reason, many are anxious to participate in the planning process that leads to community training or extended technical assistance. Only through planning can the comments be made that they feel will lead to appropriate training topics. This issue is further complicated when we realize that what the service deliverer will request and respond to depends in part on where he perceives himself at a given point in time. For example, many of those beginning their work as Title VII project directors were most concerned that training sessions cover material needed to begin a program, such as regulations, meal delivery, participant recruitment, and staff development. Only after these components were well in place were the directors interested in the process of aging, motivation, communication, and other aging-related topics. Although the latter material is equally important to an effective Title VII program, it was not perceived as being crucial until the more functional aspects of the program were competently established. New material is accepted in stages, and understanding what components are appropriate to what stage of program development and worker development is essential. Community workers have a strong sense of where they are and what they feel they need to hear.

In addition, many workers feel a strong need to be a part of the training planning because of other issues they are protecting or developing. Training might be seen as a vehicle to reinforce staff positions or build new staff relationships. Educational groups should be sensitive to the staff issues generated through training or technical assistance programs.

Fourth, those in the community usually perceive research differently from those in a university setting. Service workers are looking for new information to help them carry out tasks with more skill. They want the information as quickly and efficiently as possible. The majority of professionals have a good understanding of the importance of research in the advancement of knowledge and how it can be of value to them in their work. However, when asked to participate in research projects, or to help find subjects, they are anxious to understand what the research is about, why it would be of value to them, and how they might be able to apply it to their work once the research is completed. Frustration with participating in research projects is particularly noticeable when results are not shared and/or not generalizable enough to be implemented following the project. Community workers become reluctant to continue their involvement in research studies when they don't see what they can get in return for the efforts extended. Impatience with research methodology can also inhibit full cooperation with a project.

Fifth, sometimes there is a misunderstanding about costs, fee charges, and payment schedules. Agencies that do not incorporate funding for outside consulting have some difficulty understanding the fee structure of the university and of the faculty associated with the university. It is important that those from the university who work with community groups on joint projects involving money explain the university and/or faculty financial requirements so that the community group can understand why certain fees are charged. Much training that colleges and universities do is on a self-support basis, a point that can be easily missed by service workers. When not openly discussed, it can lead to unexpressed resentment later on.

A related matter is whether the training dollars go to those community professionals and organizations seeking training and technical assistance or whether community training dollars should go directly to the academic institutions. Since control of dollars means control of program it is important to understand that the community's interest in controlling the training dollar is one of assuring that it develops a program most closely related to what it feels it needs. It is difficult to assess and define the "real" training needs as perceived by different community and educational groups.

Both educational institutions and the community have the same goals: to find and deliver an improved quality of life to the older person. The ultimate goal is similar. It is the intermediate goals that define the uniqueness of the service. In order for universities and colleges to achieve their goals of teaching, training, research, and community technical assistance, there are important roles that the community can play. Because of what the community can offer, it is important that the universities facilitate better cooperation and understanding with community workers and organizations.

1. The community can offer a working knowledge of programs and older people. The community can offer examples of theory in action, implementation of federal legislation and regulations, and case examples of those receiving services.

2. The community can offer consultants to the university and other community groups, consultants who can share the working knowledge based on their long experience.

3. Students come from the community to university and college programs. Many students entering the field are those who have had some work experience in the field and who want to return to school to strengthen their knowledge base. College support and visibility in the community will be subtle encouragement for those wanting to return to school.

4. The community can offer support for a project, added resources, letters of support for a proposal, political muscle, and dissemination avenues for results.

5. The community can employ the graduates of educational programs and provide placements for students in school.

Without an understanding of community programs and community needs, and without support to community activity, the university or college cannot carry out its own educational functions in the field of gerontology.

The University Perspective

Because many gerontologists working in universities combine two almost independent approaches, they do not always see the conflict between these two approaches, let alone the conflicts between either approach and the community that encompasses the older people whom they seek to observe and for whom they try to promote a better life. It is only after a series of confusing confrontations that they come to understand the basic dilemma.

Present-day universities are Janus-like institutions. On the one hand, they represent the academic-scholarly tradition of questioning accepted "facts" in the service of increasing knowledge of humankind and the world in which it lives. On the other hand, they have gotten into the business of "training," a business which ignores possible questions and alternative strategies and gets down to simplified "how to's." It is interesting that most of the discussions at the Tucson meeting of AGHE—both formal and informal—centered almost completely upon the second face. The university representatives gathered there were interested almost exclusively in the training aspect and in the issues which were outlined above. They wanted guidelines, often in true "how to" fashion, for facilitating their training and "research" in the "community." And the research they were talking about was the evaluation of programs or assessment of immediate needs rather than the questioning of what programs were for, what variation there might be in needs, or what covert or progressive processes in man and society might underlie manifest need statements and make them trivial or dangerous foundations for social action.

The activist side of academic gerontologists tends to be highly sensitive to the attitudes and incidental behaviors of the workers in the field and tries to direct their teaching first of all to the confrontation with and diminution of age biases. While they recognize the desires of community workers to be stroked for their sacrificing and "dirty" work with old people—as they have been informed—they may be disturbed by the fact that those people who are "taking care" of older men and women see this work as sacrificing and dirty. They may thus try hard to increase person-to-person communication between worker and client and to break down stereotyped attitudes and prejudices about the old that prevent such communication.

The academic side of academic gerontologists is even more disturbed by workers who say they are not interested in general information about aging —biological, psychological, social or other—that they just want to be given a set of skills. How can we hand out bags of tricks when we don't know what any particular older person wants or requires? Variability is great, and programs designed for one group may be insulting or boring or deadly to another.

In this discussion, we have purposely exaggerated the perspectives of both the community and the university to point out some of the basic problems we are both facing. From an academic point of view, only when we see the nature of the problem can we start to suggest possible solutions.

Special Service Aspects of College and University Programs

Bonny Russell
San Jose State University

A discussion of services relating to gerontology as a part of the ongoing responsibility of universities and colleges could bring forth a list of great length. The broad dimensions of the list are a separate matter. The depth of responsibility of the university, the commitment of staff time, the allocation of finances, the allowances for volunteer activities, and the involvement in the community are all subjects for consideration. In his background paper for the 1971 White House Conference on Aging, Howard McClusky underlined the responsibility for education that continues through life:

From an educational standpoint the impressive and distinguishing characteristic of our time is that we are now living in a Learning Society. Within recent decades and at an ever increasing pace we have been arriving at a stage in societal development where learning is an essential condition for participation in the world about us and equally mandatory for advancement and personal development.

This new development is largely the result of profound and accelerating change. Change is now so pervasive that all aspects of living and all kinds and ages of people are affected. Moreover change has become so persistently continuous that for the first time in the history of mankind and even more so in the future, learning must be as continuous as change itself and inevitably lifelong in character.

*The implications of this new mandate for the entire enterprise of educa-
tion can scarcely be exaggerated. Its implications for meeting the educational
needs of Older Persons (O.P.'s) are even more far reaching and urgent. For in
the case of Older Persons change appears in a double and uniquely aggravat-
ing dimension. First there is the change in the society outside the person to
which we have already referred. But second there are changes in the life
situation itself, which because of their drastic consequences produce a kind of
"double jeopardy" for persons in the later years. Thus, if learning is an attempt
to adjust to and master change both within and without the individual and, if it
is to be relevant to his situation, any consideration of the educational needs of
the O.P. must, without compromise, confront the realities of the multiple
impact of change inherent in the life cycle which O.P.'s occupy. Such a
confrontation should result in the formulation of an educational program
markedly different from that associated with the "credential" system of formal
education in the earlier years.*

*. . . In brief it is argued that O.P.'s have a vital need for that kind of
education that will enable them to exert influence in protecting and improving
their own situation, and in contributing to the well-being of the larger society.* [1]

To be effective, this new kind of education should be based on the
characteristics of the older person in the learning situation. Experiments in
laboratories have demonstrated the delusive nature of those myths which
reinforce the stereotype regarding the older person's inability to learn and
adapt. If we accept the challenge of producing this service and we recognize
that there are special needs, then a service component has been added to
education programs at all levels. The universities and colleges have a large
stake in this because they are responsible for providing the professional
educator, as well as the career specialist, in the field of aging. Colleges and
universities are also major shapers of attitudes.

Should There Be Academic Programs for Older People Within the Universities and Colleges?

Many schools are seeking answers to this question today. In California a
study of Higher Education for Aging was completed in 1975. Two state
universities, San Jose and Long Beach, were selected, after legislative action,
to waive fees for students over 60. This effort was to last for a trial period of two
years. All students were to meet the same admission requirements and no
special courses could be developed for this new segment of the student body.
The number of older students admitted has been restricted to 200 on a space
available basis for each of the universities during the trial period. At San Jose
about half of this number has registered during the first year. Experiential
backgrounds of these new students (at San Jose) are varied. A fairly large group
had been teachers. Others have come from business, engineering, and social
work. Their purposes for reentering school also varied. A medical secretary

wanted an education in the field of gerontology in order to work with older people. A retired librarian was continuing a previously unfulfilled interest in mathematics. A recent widow wanted to learn business management. An engineer was moving toward a second career in psychological counseling. Still others wanted to complete their education and to obtain the degree they didn't have time for earlier, while some wanted life enrichment.

At this point in the program there seems to be a great deal of success accompanying it. The older students are almost unanimous in their praise of it. Students and faculty find that interesting discussions take place in classes because of the background knowledge and experience of the older students.

Questions that arise have to do with the need for a specially designed orientation program based on the learning characteristics of the older student. This would alleviate the problems that may exist at reentry into a learning situation. It would also provide information about the university and its programs.

There is no real question about the university's responsibility to include qualified older people in academic programs. As numbers of older people increase within our population, and as society attempts to meet the needs of a lengthened life span for more people, it must also attempt to meet the needs of greater life space. Education is an obvious vehicle through which this may be accomplished and through which quality may be added to quantity.

Should There Be Special Programs
for Older Adults?

Another aspect of education for older adults in which the university has some responsibility relates to education for living in the later years. Aging is influenced by the changing activities and patterns of society. These are both individual and social challenges. There are organic and mental changes as well as situational ones associated with aging. These require adjustments. They may also offer the elderly person new opportunities or loss of opportunities. Development of self is prerequisite to having satisfactory interaction with the changes that occur as the culture evolves and as individual life situations are altered with age. It is incumbent upon society to elevate the kinds and quality of services available to those who have not developed the ability to care for themselves, and to provide the educational tools with which the older people can maximize and utilize their own potential for continued useful participation. In discussing education for the later years at a meeting at the University of Nebraska in 1971, Carroll Londoner stated (in his paper "Enriching the Lives of Older People"):

There is a special need for programs which provide opportunities for helping older adults make life style adjustments necessary for survival. Through the adult portion of the life span one has had to develop a set of competencies in the various roles and tasks of his life. Typically, this competency is measured in terms of a person's effectiveness in his judgments and in the wise use of his skills as he meets the challenges of the various adult roles and tasks. The older adult, too, must continue to cultivate his competencies and effectiveness as he faces the challenges of old age.

In order to assist the cultivation of these competencies, the university must do more than provide education that focuses on more efficient functioning, either in work roles or in adjustment to nonwork. It must respond through providing education pertinent to lifelong needs. This education should imply the process of continuing learning for the development of the person. It should minimize any negative effect regardless of the work-nonwork dichotomy, and disassociate itself from the need for societal production efficiency. This education proposes to cause change within the individual, making him more aware, more conscious of the world in which he lives. It provides training of the mind for enjoyment, for leisure. It may incorporate information within the cultural context that will provide a basis for dealing with future crises when past solutions are no longer adequate. The many preretirement programs would also fall within this area.

Education or training can provide new knowledge for low income or minority elderly who may need assistance in learning how to cope with contemporary problems at a survival level or to provide them with information concerning available service delivery systems. Additionally, for long-term gain, it may be necessary to present education with the purpose of elevating confidence to counteract the "poor" self-image that is commonly held by older persons. Persons confident of self, aware of the surrounding world and of available options are not easily labeled poor nor easily relegated to a less than standard existence.

Some university and college services will center their activities around short-term training programs. This responsibility is very difficult to avoid because of continuous requests for such services. If the university wishes to relate effectively to the community, to receive support, financial or social, or if it wishes to use the resources of the community for its students, it must communicate its interest through action. Short-term training programs are varied and each one needs different packaging to reach the clientele it is meant to serve. Some may be related to participation of the elders in a community organizational program; others may focus on advocacy or citizenship responsibility. With the added numbers of older voters this focus may not be taken lightly.

Several colleges and universities have followed the example set earlier by the New School for Social Research in New York by establishing a separate unit as a part of the school in which older people, with interest in education, develop their own institute and curriculum tailored to meet the wishes and needs of the group. Funding has been varied, and fees, grants, and donations have been used to underwrite the programs. Examples include University of California Extension Services program in San Francisco, C.L.I.R. (Center for Learning in Retirement), and the Fromm Institute of the University of San Francisco. There are many others.

Community colleges' very successful efforts in behalf of older people have included the organization of college-community committees to develop special events, emeritus groups, special courses to address the needs of older people, and the use of these committees to recruit older people in the continuing program of the colleges. In some areas the numbers of mature people registered reach as high as 70 percent in the extended day programs.

Of the accepted services available for use by the community, including a large group of older people, are public lectures, concerts, theater presentations, museum displays, and athletic events. Some universities have taken further steps, serving both the elderly and the students through establishing senior centers on or near campus, by opening cafeterias during non-rush hours, or by opening swimming pools when they are not otherwise being used. Housing projects for older people have been established on campuses along with housing for students. These provide excellent opportunities for student training in several occupations such as housing administrators, food operators, or program directors for multipurpose senior centers.

Education for Professionals
in the Field of Aging

There is no question about the responsibility of universities in providing adequate education for professionals in the field of aging. This responsibility may also be expanded to include providing education for professionals who have "transferred" to this field with no academic education in it or for paraprofessionals who are most often older persons working in community programs for seniors. Because there are continuing changes in gerontology and in the governmental laws and regulations concerning organization of programs, it is highly important that such individuals be provided with the opportunity to become aware of and to learn about new developments. Some universities have endeavored to meet the needs of these practitioners by developing a credential program with a required number of units in gerontology. There are usually no prerequirements for this program because their purpose is to upgrade the level of education in gerontology for as many workers as possible.

University Involvement in Community Activities

Because community projects for seniors are frequently used for students' field placements, it is essential for the well-being of the university programs that continuing relationships be established in the community. These relationships also provide university programs with opportunities to use the community as its field in research projects and to provide student volunteers with roles in community programs. It is important that educators are interested and able to find the best combination of school and community experiences for educational purposes. Educators may also find it worthwhile to establish relationships in the community for continuing knowledge of growth and changes, for use of developing resources, and for awareness of attitudinal changes.

An interesting concept was underwritten with Title III, Older Americans Act funds in California when Senior Californian Education Centers were established. Joint grants were made available to cities and universities or colleges to establish a center in which each would have a specific role. Through these grants, opportunities were made available in two areas: (1) to increase community awareness and involvement in the problems of older people, and (2) to continue to assist the older person to function independently as part of his community. Through a designated department, the city's role included expansion and analysis of service and activity programs. The university's role included planning, establishing, and coordinating curricula for four groups: professionals working with older people, community groups and agencies including civic leaders and volunteers, students, and older persons.

Serving on boards of community organizations, participating as planners and speakers at seminars and meetings, speaking for service clubs, providing information on various subjects to community organizations or industry, testifying at city council meetings are all important in establishing an ongoing relationship for the university and the community. Often these involvements can be seriously time consuming and therefore each request for such activity should be considered carefully and choices made in relation to their importance to university goals.

Another community related university activity is to assist in the evaluation of community programs for older people. Time involved in such things as the development and application of the evaluation instrument or materials may be overwhelming for the individuals doing these things, but the advantages to older persons in the programs being evaluated and to future programs far outweigh the cost in effort or dollars.

Universities are frequently called upon to develop curriculum or teaching materials for in-service training programs for organizations serving the older population. If one of the goals of the university is to help in the provision of more effective staff and better services for older people then this is an important service.

Where possible, the university should also provide service to the community through its research activities and particularly through the interpretation or translation of pertinent research data for immediate use in appropriate program activities. Research utilization can enhance present programs and set future standards. Community suggested research projects should be thoroughly evaluated and considered favorably if they have meaning both for the university and the community.

The publication of pamphlets, proceedings of institutes, books, and articles addressing the needs of older people is of major importance as a service of universities and colleges. This enables information to be communicated as it becomes available; as a result there is a deeper understanding of problems and solutions and new and effective endeavors in the field are stimulated.

It may seem that this paper has delivered a "laundry list" and not the laundry. But, if there is to be the laundry—a total program of services by the university or college—then it is essential that universities work together. Forces must be joined on each campus. An interdisciplinary and comprehensive approach must be maintained to bring understanding about aging to all college staff. This interdisciplinary group must interface with the community group to engage in planning, coordinating and establishing coalitions, to the end that roles are clear, funds are available, and services meet the needs as they arise and that university and college planning and services dovetail with the planning and services of the community.

Note

1. Howard Y. McClusky, *Education: Background and Issue Papers to the 1971 White House Conference on Aging*, pp. 1 and 5.

Issues in Education for Older Adults

Vivian Wood
University of Wisconsin

The workshop relating to issues in education for older adults was designed to deal with issues in three areas:

1. Why?
    - Need for special programs for older adults
    - Is there a real demand
    - Reason for widespread and rapid development
2. What?
    - Types of programs in existence
    - Purposes/needs they are serving
    - What types of colleges can best do what
    - What is a quality program
3. For whom?
    - Who is participating, who is not
    - Who bears the cost and why
    - What types of programs do older adults really want

While designed to deal with all these issues, in reality only part of them were considered, and in varying degrees. It was pointed out that the growth of mandatory retirement at lower ages is related to the growing pool of potential postretirement students available to participate in higher education. It is important to consider the purposes of education at this phase of life. The reader is cautioned to "resist the shoddy and the easy." We need to remember that the kind of education we provide is a function of our perceptions of life as a whole. We need to be concerned about the quality of educational programming for older adults. All too often some educational institutions offer "golden age garbage."

A report entitled "Continuing Education for the Elderly: A Report of a Conference at Dominican College, Ohio" (December, 1976) containing information on program planning for older adults in higher education was distributed. Some time was spent outlining a framework for viewing education for older adults developed by Dr. H. R. Moody, Hunter College, entitled "Philosophical Presuppositions of Education for Old Age" (1976). Dr. Moody, a philosopher, was in the audience and contributed to the discussion.

Moody's thesis is that education for the older adult, unlike education for the young, is not functionally required for the maintenance of society and, accordingly, has low priority. We have no clear purposes or principles on which to base educational programs for older adults. He presented four sets of societal attitudes that have guided and continue to guide the development of educational programs. He views these modal patterns as stages through which societies pass in their treatment of the elderly, each of which has implications for education.

Briefly, the four modal patterns are: (1) rejection—no educational opportunities provided; (2) social services—older adults viewed as consumers for whom entertainment-oriented or "keep 'em busy" courses are provided; (3) participation—older adults demand autonomy and roles in the mainstream of society; education is for second careers and leadership roles; and (4) self-actualization—education in philosophy, religion, literature, and psychology encourages spiritual and humanistic growth. Our society is seen to be at the social services stage with some groups such as the Gray Panthers trying to move older adults into the participation mode.

It was pointed out that Moody's self-actualization stage is something of an ideal because: (a) a substantial proportion of today's older population has had little or no basic education; (b) the majority of older people are women, many of whom, in raising a family and maintaining a home, had little time for intellectual pursuits and who grew up when education for women was often considered a waste; and (c) many older adults grew up at a time when being old enough to quit school was an eagerly awaited event.

Issue: Should the goal of education for all older adults be the same? Alternatively, if we follow the principle of taking the student from where he is, do we have the capabilities for accomplishing this with adults who start from many different levels?

Some of the most educationally deprived persons in our society are in the 65 and older age group. *Issue*: Should education for older adults be a right to which they are entitled? The "audit-only-as-space-is-available" policy of many universities is an indication that education as a right is not widely accepted. A workshop participant quoted an older student: "I don't want to audit life—I want to take it for credit."

Dr. Wood presented data on a University of Wisconsin-Madison study which indicated that interest in attending the University was very low among older adults in the community. *Issue*: How much effort should be made to motivate older adults to go to school? *Issue*: How much of education for older adults should take place through higher education?

Workshop participants raised many issues to which no easy answers are available. There was consensus, however, that education for older adults is an area in which there will be widespread activity and development in the next decade.

Reference

Moody, H. R. Philosophical presuppositions of education for old age. *Educational Gerontology*, 1976, *1*, 1–16.

Section Five

Introduction to Administration:
General or Unique

The administration of multidisciplinary problems in discipline-based universities can often try people's souls. Administration of gerontology programs may also be complicated by the "soft money-hard money" support system. The papers in this section comment on some of the perils of such administration.

The Sweet Smell of Money— The Misguided Motivation?

Ellen Page Robin
Western Michigan University

If we assume that the availability of money may create misguided motivation and its absence leave motivation pristine, then I know I was invited to be on this program because I have had program money briefly and have been without it for a much longer time. The relationship of money-availability to the quality of motivation is not so clear-cut as our title suggests. We have worked to develop a gerontology program at Western Michigan University since 1969. Courses were introduced in 1970. The program—an undergraduate minor—was fully operational in the spring of 1975. We received our first training grant in the summer of 1976. In candor, I have to say that we had applied a number of times prior to this. In candor also I have to admit that it's considerably more comfortable being relatively rich than absolutely poor.

My plan is to look briefly at some of the pitfalls of academic planning by grant availability; I will not spend a great deal of time with these as we have all thought about and heard them before. I would like to talk about what can be done without grant money because much can be and has been accomplished in this condition.

First, let us discuss the pitfalls of grants—for gerontology as well as other areas of academic concern. Academic planning is not a process which should be stimulated solely by the availability of grant money. Academic planning should be based on a thorough knowledge of the strengths and goals of the institution and its constituent parts. If grant availability and the strengths and goals of the institution mesh, then certainly desired results can be accomplished more readily and rapidly with funding than without. Further, if the desired goals include development of faculty competence in a particular area, hiring new faculty having the desired interests, education, and skills with outside funding is a more thorough and rapid a method than are others. If, however, academic planning follows money, the institution may be littered with reminders and remainders of academic fads for which money has dried up, with programs which must remain of questionable quality for want of adequately prepared and adequately supported faculty and staff, with students ill-prepared to meet the challenges of the fields they have chosen (if the fields exist any more), and finally, an institution whose educational focus is blurred and confused by this educational debris.

Grant money is notoriously unpredictable. You cannot count on its coming your way even if you're sure that your institutional goals meet agency priorities. Further, once granted, there are no guarantees today that it will continue beyond the grant year. If all the institutional program hopes rest in the *funded* program, they may be just as uncertain and short-lived as the funding. Particularly difficult here are: (1) the dashed hopes of the staff who have spent so much time and have invested so much energy in planning and carrying out the program—as far as it went; (2) potential unemployment of those faculty hired on soft money for this program—if the institution cannot or will not pick it up. One can speak of the moral responsibility of the institution all one wishes, but if a state of financial crisis exists—as it truly does in many institutions—or even relative paucity of funds and if the money is not there, then it cannot be spent to save a program which has lost its funding.

One way to assure greater institutional commitment and support is to build all of the academic instructional components of the proposed program on hard money. Hard-money programs are those which rest on institutional commitment. If the program is important—and gerontology programs are important to students, faculty, institutions, and the local, state, and national communities—then institutional commitment is important to initiate, build, and maintain. In part, here, we substitute hard work and time for money—a traditional trade-off—but one which has become increasingly rare. A base of hard-money support becomes a firm foundation for grant money expansion of program, for developing and expanding research efforts, and for community services. But it is frequently a difficult task. How to accomplish this?

A seemingly obvious but overlooked first step is to determine the current level of interest in gerontology on the campus. Faculty and departmental surveys often turn up interest in the most unexpected places and reading catalogue course descriptions may yield a number of existing courses and/or parts of courses which are particularly relevant to an academic program in gerontology. (A note of warning here—don't count on department chairpersons or deans or other spokespersons to know course description content. They often don't. Don't substitute the survey for reading of the catalogue—

faculty who do not consider themselves knowledgeable of or particularly interested in gerontology may be teaching perfectly appropriate courses for your purposes.) Make the faculty and catalogue survey a regular event— interests change and so do courses. A human benefit of this process is to bring together persons of like interests who may not have known of each other's existence. A political benefit is to make the survey-maker a focus of gerontological activity, a rallying point in the present and future.

Establish a planning committee under appropriate aegis. If you are thinking in terms of a single department containing the contemplated academic program, then the department chair could provide the necessary clout. If multidisciplinary, but within a single college, a dean would be appropriate. If your known and projected faculty interests extend beyond the boundaries of a single college, your home might logically be directly under the president, provost, or vice president for academic affairs. This is an ideal place, by the way, as it tends to remove you from departmental jealousies and from the political and, perhaps, fiscal maneuverings of hard-pressed academic deans. A rule of thumb is to secure the support of the highest placed administrator appropriate to the unit placement of the program.

The committee should be prepared to decide, in a preliminary way, the design of the desired programs, to compare the current level of development with the goals to determine development needs and priorities, and to begin to move to develop necessary faculty competence and/or courses. In times of financial need, programs which largely are new combinations of existing interests and courses are more economical and more likely to win supporters. Further, the committee needs to develop visibility within the university/ college community. This visibility will call attention to the interest in gerontology both on and off campus and will make it somewhat easier to have new courses approved, to attract students, to shift the balance of interest toward this new program.

What can be done? How about a preretirement series for faculty and staff? Personnel departments are usually happy to cooperate in such a program and can suggest and/or supply many resource people—chiefly in the financial aspects of retirement—for such a program. (Certainly people need to plan more than the financial aspects of their retirement, but if this is a first effort, you'll find them more interested in the financial aspects than any other. You can always add other topics—leisure time use, continuing professional involvement, housing, estate planning—at a later series.)

The committee should make known to its members and to all other interested faculty and staff all opportunities for further development of professional competence through courses, workshops, relevant organizations' memberships and/or meetings.

A survey of library and audiovisual holdings provides support services to a faculty hard-pressed for time—and also provides a basis for requesting a greater part of those budgets to be spent in acquisition of gerontological materials. In the meantime and within current library and audiovisual budgets, request such acquisitions. These requests may lead to acquisitions and will certainly make your interests known to library and audiovisual staff.

A regional survey of occupational needs and employment opportunities in gerontology serves several functions. It provides those within the institution responsible for enrollment the promise of immediate payoff. It creates a guide for the committee in the addition of new courses and other program development. It gives the program added visibility outside the institution. It helps to place graduates of the program, an inestimable help for a fledgling effort. And, it serves as a basis for any external request for funding you might want to make in the future.

The addition of courses to the existing curriculum should be planned as carefully as possible based on your knowledge of your university or college procedures. If courses can be added first in the most hospitable department(s), this strategy may make course additions elsewhere more easily accomplished. All course additions, however, should proceed on the basis of your ultimate vision and should, hopefully, have a reasoned place in the program-to-be.

Become visible in community service in those programs serving or planning for older citizens. In this way, your interests and programs become known. People and community programs seeking help will turn to you—making your efforts still more visible; students needing field placements and, ultimately, jobs will find a more hospitable welcome from those who have followed and benefited from your development. I regard continuing education as a community service and have seen the accrual of many benefits from taking our courses into the surrounding portions of the state.

Now for the ultimate ingredient in any academic program—students. Gerontologists, as others, have been known to accept usual community views of old age and old people and have thought it necessary to purchase student participation in programs dealing with such topics. Much of the early support to gerontological programs in universities went to purchase such student interest. If this was ever necessary, it is not at present—at least from the experience at my institution and others of which I have knowledge. Our courses consistently fill. The numbers of students in our program have multiplied and we have student *demand* for a graduate component which we shall add in the fall of 1977. In notifying students of the availability of your program and in recruiting them, it is of paramount importance not to promise more than can be delivered. We cannot mislead students about the availability of jobs—but we can help them learn to sell their skills to potential employers.

I think, however, of at least two circumstances in which payment to students more than pays off: (1) We currently have 10 undergraduate assistants in gerontology (each working five hours per week for a faculty member—for the grand sum of $165 per semester). This part of our program has had enormous results—it has stimulated course and research development among the faculty; it has provided undergraduate students with faculty contacts they would never have had; and has provided educational experiences otherwise unavailable. (2) In graduate programs especially, the stimulation of research efforts among faculty and students is of major concern and priority. The ability to provide research assistantships facilitates research efforts and there is no substitute here for the money needed to purchase necessary time.

If you are successful in building your program on a solid base of hard money, the addition of grant money is less likely to swamp your program since those monies will be sought and be used to *supplement* your existing program rather than *shape* it. Of course, new components may be added, but they are less likely to mold your goals or change your direction. Further, if you are successful in seeking funds but unsuccessful at keeping them on a long-term basis, the loss of funding, while perhaps a major inconvenience and disappointment, will not destroy your program.

One final word—beware of funding success. Enjoy it, certainly, but be wary of the sense of security it provides. Use it to develop your program in the ways you have communally decided are most reasonable and needed, but avoid overreaching your scarce commodities of time, talent, and commitment. Above all, when requesting funds and receiving them, always plan for their possible termination—decide contingency plans in advance and avoid dependency.

Perils of Program Administration

Carter C. Osterbind
University of Florida

I think the editors have entitled this section "Perils of Program Administration" to stress those aspects of administering gerontological programs that create the greatest road-blocks to their successful implementation. Thus our focus is on the types of major problems that may be inevitable in the development of gerontological programs within a college or university. One of the great values of coming together as representatives of educational institutions in an organization such as this is that we exchange views, not about textbook type or even an ivory-towered, removed-from-the-real-world type of situation, but rather we bring to these discussions the real problems that we are facing from day to day in the development of the type of program each of us represents. I am director of a multidisciplinary center at the University of Florida, and we have engaged in the development of what we have termed a four-phase program. I would like to outline the program plan because it has relevance to the problems I will discuss and it may also suggest other matters that should be brought out in the workshop.

In 1950, a university-wide committee designated as the Council for the Institute of Gerontology was appointed by the president of the University of Florida. This committee established the Institute of Gerontology (renamed the Center for Gerontological Studies and Programs in 1971). The main function of the Institute was to hold an Annual Southern Conference on

Gerontology. The purpose of the Conference was to bring together professionals and others interested in the problems of aging. In 1973 a major change occurred. Now the Center for Gerontological Studies and Programs is in the second two-year phase of an eight-year program planned in 1973–74 to develop a multidisciplinary gerontology center at the University of Florida. The Center program when fully developed will cover undergraduate, graduate, and professional education and include programs in continuing education, research, and public service. The program is based on the finding that there is a need for it and that there are extensive resources in the University that are already committed to gerontology and others that may be drawn upon for the program. The general schedule for all four phases of the Center program is set out below.

◆ Phase I (1973–74 and 1974–75). (1) Obtain commitments of support from key administrators in the University and State University System; (2) develop interest and activity by existing faculty in research and teaching in gerontology; (3) add courses in gerontology to existing curriculums; (4) bring in new faculty interested in gerontology; (5) continue to work on plans for extension of programs; (6) obtain additional support for programs.

◆ Phase II (1975–76 and 1976–77). Develop a multidisciplinary graduate program that will provide gerontological content to graduate degree programs in sociology, psychology, architecture, communications, counseling, education, economics, and planning, and foster multidisciplinary research and service projects in gerontology.

◆ Phase III (1977–78 and 1978–79). Extend the graduate program into other areas and add gerontological content in law, medicine, and other professional areas. Implement a summer program in 1977 and develop it in additional areas in 1978. Plan and develop an undergraduate program in social gerontology.

◆ Phase IV (1979–80 and 1980–81). Develop specialty undergraduate programs with gerontological content.

You can see from this brief review of the four-phase program that we have been moving from a highly specialized, limited type of program that had focused principally on developing more effective communications between those interested in gerontology to a highly diversified one involving a major commitment of university resources.

In stressing the perils faced in administering our program, I will give attention to the following topics: (1) funding, (2) accounting practices and administrative procedures, (3) curriculum development, (4) staffing, (5) program evaluation, and (6) the prerogatives of the Center. I will not give exhaustive discussion of each subject, but rather illustrate the nature of particular problems and thus lay the basis for our more detailed discussion of them.

1. Funding

The most difficult problem we face is securing a stable and adequate source of funding that will enable us to develop programs in an efficient, cost-effective way. A major part of this problem is that of redirecting and obtaining control over funds that are available within the institution itself. This means that there is the continuing problem of working with a number of administrative groups—colleges and professional schools, departments within those colleges, other centers and research groups, and individuals in a variety of programs—and getting them to commit resources to the center program. For example, if there is a desire to utilize funding from sources over which the center has no direct administrative control, it is necessary to get commitments from the various departments and professional schools to carry forward instructional or other types of support on a continuing and stable basis. Thus, in building the funding base of the center, it becomes important to gradually build a wellspring of support from within the university. We can expand on this in the course of the discussion.

Another problem associated with funding is the difficulty of getting funds for purposes that are consistent with the central thrust of the center program. Quite frequently, there are conditions attached to funding that require specific types of programs or research to be carried out. This creates problems when these programs are undertaken and must be integrated with existing programs and the outside funding utilized in a manner that will result in the most productive development of all programs. It is true, also, that once a program gets under way, the opportunity to secure funds for activities that are not closely related, or which are somewhat diversionary in terms of carrying out the objectives of the broader program, arises, and it becomes necessary to determine if funds for those purposes should be sought, or should be foregone and efforts directed at other opportunities. It is also difficult to determine the most fruitful avenues to pursue when there is a limitation on time and manpower for seeking funds. Quite frequently, it is not clear which course to pursue, and it appears necessary to pursue multiple options when it would be much better if these efforts could be restricted.

Another aspect of funding that creates problems pertains to the limitations on the use of grant funds. Quite frequently, funds are available for one of our unmet program needs, but because of specific limitations on how the funds may be used, they impose problems that impede the effective development of the program. One example of this is the restrictions imposed on grant funds for student support. Unless the funds are available on a basis which allows effective competition with other scholarships, it is not possible to bring the best qualified students into the program.

2. Accounting Practices and Administrative Procedures

One of the biggest problems which we are continually confronting at the

University of Florida, and I know it is a widespread one, pertains to the inflexibility in the discretionary use of funds because of accounting procedures and regulations. It becomes difficult to transfer funds that have been allocated to one specific function to another function. For example, to transfer salary funds to expense, or to transfer student support funds to salary funds or to capital outlay funds. These constraints, which are imposed in part by accounting procedures and in part by the terms of grants, quite often result in the very inefficient use of funds. Another problem is the procedural red tape that results from accounting regulations and administrative procedures. I know it is true at the University of Florida, and elsewhere, that the requirements for approvals of all types create serious constraints on the effective utilization of time and on program implementation. For example, at the University of Florida, there is a wide diversity both in accounting practices and administrative procedures among the different colleges and departments that are involved in the center program. If I wish to buy the time of a staff member directly from a grant or a contract, the procedures to be followed and benefits of this to a particular department or to the individual involved vary greatly, depending upon the policies that exist within the department or college. Quite frequently the university implements some broad general policies but allows exceptions at the college and departmental levels. These exceptions create obstacles that can be dealt with only by skill and unlimited patience.

3. Curriculum Development

In a large university the multidisciplinary nature of gerontology creates problems in curriculum development. First, there are the generally recognized turf problems. A course in counseling may be taught by those in educational counseling, psychology, clinical psychology, or in some other subject area that has credentials for teaching counseling. In a multidisciplinary program, there are many types of instruction that cut across the traditional disciplines and professional areas and raise questions as to who is the professional or educator most qualified to deal with aspects of the subject. Associated with development and administration of curriculum are content selection and priority problems that exist within each department and college, and which must be confronted in terms of a variety of considerations. There are also the procedural problems associated with established committee structures in the university. Each department has its curriculum committee; each college has its curriculum committee; the undergraduate educational programs have curriculum committees; the graduate programs have curriculum committees; the professional schools have curriculum committees and accrediting agencies; all of these committees interact and create a broad range of problems that must be coped with successfully if the best type of curriculum is to be developed and the best type of staff committed to teaching the curriculum.

4. Staffing

In a multidisciplinary center the staff can be employed solely by the center, solely by the administrative units associated with the center, or by both. The second approach is being followed in the main at the University of Florida, and we think that it is a sound one, but it is not without problems. It becomes necessary to develop strategies that will make it possible to bring into departments outstanding people in the particular departmental field who have a strong commitment to gerontology and will develop a departmental commitment to gerontology that is consistent with educational goals of the center. The particular strategies that we have followed and the problems these present will be a part of our discussion.

5. Program Evaluation

I believe that one of the fears of many who operate programs in gerontology is that the program will be evaluated by someone who is not qualified to do so. The lack of qualifications may be assumed to exist because the evaluator is from another discipline or professional area. It is obvious that if a program is interdisciplinary in nature, the peer group of evaluators could be a rather diverse group. It is often difficult to know who is qualified within these peer groups to make judgments in areas such as law, architecture, the humanities, the behavioral and social and hard sciences, and in the professions of nursing, medicine, etc. The evaluation must take into account the way in which gerontology fits into the many programs of which it is a part, and conversely it must consider the way in which these programs fit into gerontology. I like to think that in making the evaluations, the one common criterion is the ultimate objective of obtaining superior educational programs and experiences for students. There is so much knowledge to impart that selection and compromise must be central concerns.

6. The Prerogatives of the Center

There are the problems associated with an identification of the true function and role of a center in the university. At the University of Florida, we have many types of centers. Some of these centers are restricted to a particular discipline or professional area, frequently are essentially within a department, and focus on the special interests of a department. There are centers that house the research or other types of functions within a professional school or a discipline, and there are centers that purport to be university-wide in their activity. The Center for Gerontological Studies and Programs at the University of Florida is designed to be university-wide, and thus it must cope with all of the problems that this breadth involves if the thrust of the center is to be truly a university thrust. In other words, our goal is to provide a central point for planning and coordinating all programs within the University of Florida that are in any way related to aging. In some instances the pursuit of programs in this context seems simple, in others most complex. Therefore time must be given on a continuing basis to a delineation of the prerogatives of the center within the context of the support which the center receives and opposition it encounters within the university.

I have presented some rather general ideas, hoping that these will form the basis on which we can exchange views and raise questions that will be beneficial to all of us. As I indicated in my initial comments, I have discussed some of the problems we have at the University of Florida, but obviously this does not preclude discussion of these topics from the other points of view, nor should this restrict the topics of the workshop.

Perils of Program Administration

Martin B. Loeb
University of Wisconsin

I once worked in a building in Berkeley that used to be a Unitarian Seminary. Over the door, carved in marble, were the words in Latin, "Non administrare sed administrari." Now I think that means, "Do not administrate, but be ministered to." A crazy thought at best, and a guide of caution at worst.

The major peril of program administration is to do too much of it—so that, in positive terms, do as little as possible. As you shall read, I intend to let you in on the secrets of *non administrare*.

Let me start by telling you that all the research of the vaunted Harvard Business School confirms that there is no way of managing scientifically. Any administrator can, and should, call on the body of knowledge about human behavior—remember though, we really don't know any more about human behavior today than we did many thousands of years ago. Our knowledge is in different form, conceptualized and often cauterized, but it can be useful.

Whatever knowledge is available tends to get converted into some sort of ready usefulness which we call technology. In administration, there is lots of use of technology.

Technology is one thing, but technique is another. Some people try to technologize technique; two of the most famous of these are Ben Spock in his book on *Baby and Child Care* and that other how-to book by a famous gerontologist called *The Joy of Sex*, which has been a great Comfort to many people, including the author.

I will confine my remarks to untechnologized techniques used to reduce the perils of program administration.

Now the perils are mostly not seeing to it that things get done which ought to be done, or which you promised to do.

Let's look at the first perilous area—*Money*. Too little money is a terrible thing, but too much money can be troublesome. When our Institute got started and people found out that a foundation was funding us, we got (and still get) requests for money. It is great to be able to say we don't have any—we are just here to help people get money from somewhere else. If we had money, we would have to make decisions which may make a few happy, and the many unhappy. Many techniques of program administration are used to keep people happy—in fact, make people love you. If you do everything right, you can get away with it. For example, if you help someone apply for money to some foundation, and he or she gets it, then you take all the credit you can milk out of the situation. If the funding is not forthcoming, then a little tenderness about how, with a little more thought and care, the next submission will be more successful.

But how to help? When talking over projects, one ought to know how to add and subtract relatively large numbers in your head—always round numbers—this is related to making quick, incisive statements about the size of the budget. It also involves knowing the salary habits of your own institution and other standard costs, as well as knowing the financing capabilities of various federal agencies and foundations. For example, small foundations want a big bang for their few bucks, whereas often the federal agencies are concerned primarily about getting you going and keeping your accounts straight. Anyway, one carries around a lot of information of an arithmetic nature that goes from salaries to federal appropriations and includes knowing numbers, like 426 or Title IX of legislation, at the local, state, and federal levels. A good administrator is number-oriented. Most are because they became administrators since they did not have much future in research, either because they were never good at it, or because they have burned out. (It is also true that the crime rate among the elderly is very low . . . criminals burn out, too.)

I propose to come back to money later, but a second peril is politics—as used by Aristotle rather than Nixon. "Man is by nature a political animal" (Aristotle, *Politics*). Or "Politics is the art of human happiness" (Herbert Albert Laurens Fisher, 1865–1940, whoever he is, *A History of Europe*). "Politics is the art of getting along with people gainfully" (Loeb, 1913—). A program administrator has to deal with federal government people—elected and appointed; state government people—elected and appointed; foundations—self-motivated; university administrators—appointed; colleagues—mutually chosen; staff—hired; spouse, etc.—contract.

So one learns to write letters and make phone calls to legislators, trade usefulnesses with government employees (scratching each other's back), understand the motivations and interests of foundations, and be overly attentive to university rules so that there are brownie points when one needs exceptions.

But then there are colleagues—the principle here is to give them a lot of say, but little power—help them coalesce (interdisciplinary) but only in small groups. Learn to make quick and firm decisions when absolutely necessary, otherwise use the principle of calculated delay.

There is the principle of delegation of power upwards—that is, you pass along responsibility by saying as accurately as possible, "You can do this better than I." But then there is the notion of leadership which often means giving suggestions to those to whom you have delegated power.

You are dependent on your staff. Never make an enemy of any member of your staff except by firing him or her. Instead, give them responsibility for as much as possible and a little more. Go on lots of trips so that they can get a lot of work done. Finally, in this section on politics, remember to make good trades with spouse—for every six visiting firemen one brings home for dinner, there should be one weekend at some not-too-distant motel with swimming pool or other currency.

Old people are the subject of our research and training, but in reality, money is the root of all gerontology and politics is the way you spread it around. To acquire these, one needs acumen, insensitivity, a sense of humor, and the ability to smile.

Should you want to take on program administration, you can paraphrase yourself for what I like in its pristine form from Milton's *L'Allegro*:

> *Haste thee, Nymph, and bring with thee*
> *Jest, and youthful jollity.*
> *Quips and cranks and wanton wiles,*
> *Nods and becks and wreathed smiles.*

(1631)

Or then there is the other side of the coin—for this we refer you to Rudyard Kipling and his poem, "If."

Reference

Kipling, R. *The collected works of Rudyard Kipling.* New York: Doubleday, Doran & Co., Inc., 1941.

APPENDIX:
FURTHER ISSUES IN
CURRICULUM DEVELOPMENT

Specific case studies of programs and outlines of syllabi were presented in the workshops. Details of these case studies and syllabi can be obtained directly from the presenters:

- Dr. Dana Gable, Graduate Chairman, Department of Psychology, Hood College, Frederick, Maryland: case study of Hood College's Master of Arts Program in Gerontological Counseling
- Dr. Clavin Field, Director of the Institute of Gerontology, University of the District of Columbia, Mt. Vernon Square Campus, Washington, D.C.: a case study of a Proposal for Interdisciplinary Masters Degree in Gerontology
- Dr. Ann McIver, Chairperson, Gerontology Department, Molloy College, Rockville Centre, New York: additional details on "Gerontology—A Single Discipline Model"
- Emily Miller, Librarian, Andrus Center Research and References Library, University of Southern California, Los Angeles, California: annotated sampling of existing sources in some selection tools for gerontological literature

Some papers presented at the preconference workshops and others that did not deal directly with the theme of the meetings have been included in this appendix. The authors of these papers focused on curriculum materials, providing resource information on how curricula can be developed and presented.

On Teaching the Biology of Aging

Richard C. Adelman
Temple University

The following approach to the development of a curriculum for teaching the biology of aging considers three distinct levels of examination. These include: (1) concepts and descriptive changes, (2) the pursuit of underlying molecular mechanisms, and (3) the development, maintenance and exploitation of experimental resources. Typical examples of relevant subject matter are indicated below for each of these general categories.

I. Concepts and descriptive changes
   A. Evaluation of theories of aging
   B. Genetic and environmental determinants of senescence
   C. Decline in physiological performance and its relationship to disease
   D. Cellular changes (e.g., cellular immunity)
   E. Biochemical changes (e.g., enzyme regulation)
II. Pursuit of molecular mechanisms
   A. Establishment of parameters of aging
   B. Localization of lesions within specific cell populations of particular tissues
   C. Identification of limiting biochemical events
   D. Determination of events which control the initial expression of biochemical change at a specific time in the life span
   E. Consideration of the likelihood and sociological consequences of tampering with such events

III. Experimental resources
   A. Animal models
      1. Suitability of various species
      2. Criteria for genetic and environmental maintenance
      3. Distribution for experimentation
   B. Cellular models
      1. Cultured cells derived from human tissue
      2. Cultured cells derived from species of different life spans
      3. Red blood cells
      4. Single-cell organisms
   C. Human models
      1. Cross-sectional versus longitudinal studies
      2. Ethical limitations
      3. Precocious aging syndromes

There are several possible variations on theme indicated in the above outline. All of this material currently is being prepared in the form of a practical textbook. Subsequently the major issue will concern communication between the biological and social sciences.

A Sociology of Age:
What Would It Look Like?

Beth B. Hess
County College of Morris and
Russell Sage Foundation Program on Aging

One wishes that a sociology of anything would be as simple to describe as a duck, for instance; then we could simply claim that if it waddles and quacks like a duck and looks like a duck, it must be a duck. Alas, there are as many sociologies as there are sociologists, and then some—much like the three rabbis shipwrecked on a deserted island who proceeded to establish four synagogues. I am reasonably certain that somewhere in some nursing home there is an older sociologist playing the role of a patient in an attempt to understand the existential phenomenology of patientness, or a younger researcher on the custodial staff doing an ethnomethodology of staff-patient situated encounters.

Yet another type of sociologist will be symbolically interacting with the university computer, both infinitely regressing into a world of tau, beta, lambda, and Pearsonian correlations, seeking relations of significance between, say, number of siblings and retirement income. Clearly, while both approaches can drift into silliness and even meaninglessness, each is valid sociology and has brought us many valuable insights, although I must confess being unable to understand either. Fortunately there is a broad middle area of shared theory and practice which can be fashioned into a sociology of aging appropriate and adequate for undergraduate education.

It is, as I'm sure all of you know, impossible to ignore totally a host of biological and psychological variables when studying aging, but my task is to indicate what a more or less "pure" sociology curriculum would look like. As an old-fashioned unrepentent structure-functionalist (I still call myself a political "liberal," which should indicate both old-fashionedness and unrepentence to a punishing degree), my emphasis will be on abstract social system properties. Often, when asked by students how sociology differs from social work, I reply that social workers deal with real people and we deal with ideas about people. However, the kind of intellectual distance which allows for objectivity can also become social distance permitting us to gloss over the daily reality of being old in the land of the young. With these *caveats* in mind then, let me outline what I think ought to be covered from the perspective of sociology.

One way to organize the material is to utilize the traditional triad of culture, social system, and individual as levels of analysis, within a historical framework. One could begin with a model of cultural development or evolution, which allows for cross-cultural and cross-temporal comparisons, and which specifies the unique cultural characteristics of modern industrialism. The particular paradigm that I have pieced together from various sources, and which I use when introducing any special area of sociological examination looks like this:

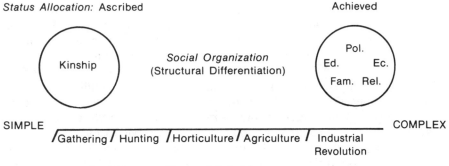

Status Allocation: Ascribed   Achieved

Kinship   *Social Organization* (Structural Differentiation)   Pol. Ed. Ec. Fam. Rel.

SIMPLE   COMPLEX

/Gathering / Hunting / Horticulture / Agriculture / Industrial Revolution

Mode of Subsistence

One can thus envisage the cumulative history of human culture as mapped along a continuum representing degrees of institutional differentiation from the polar types of simple to complex. That the complexity of societal forms is related to changes in mode of subsistence can be graphically shown. My presentation oversimplifies, of course, but that is precisely the purpose. I tend to assign causal priority to the mode of subsistence variable since this determines the size of groups able to remain together over long periods of time; and the size of the permanent population and stability of land tenure lead to division of labor, specialization of function, and ultimately, institutional differentiation out of a kinship matrix into separate areas of control and behavior. As you can easily see, the basic argument is that the development of complex societal forms gradually reduces the power of kinship-based authority and control, and that as more statuses depending upon achievement criteria open up in a society, young people are able to "liberate" themselves from family and community constraints: in mate selection, occupational choice, and voluntariness of kin-oriented relations. With the factory system the division between home and work becomes physical as well as psychological, family members turn inward to one another for emotional rather than economic needs, and generations become nucleated in all spheres.

In this fashion, we can relate the changes which take place at all three levels of analysis—cultural, societal, and individual—which would affect the position of old people in each institutional sphere: work, family, religion, education, and the polity. A course could be organized by taking up each level and looking at institutional changes affecting the aged in each sphere (Table A), or take the spheres one by one and detail the historical shifts at each level (Table B). A sociology of age must, in some fashion, deal with all this material if it is to be comprehensive and capable of articulating with other sociology courses.

To be more explicit, following Table A, if we examine each of the major areas of societal activity—those institutional spheres in which individuals have locations in patterned relationship to other status incumbents—we can see to what extent the position of old people has been undermined as a result of modernization. In the sphere of family, parental control over offspring diminishes as achievement criteria replace ascription in placing young adults in the broader social systems. Where property and family name are no longer the essential insignia of social status, lineage loses its importance. And, where relative freedom of mate choice and the ideology of romantic love characterize the marriage market, parental power and the sense of familial obligation decline. Conjugality rather than consanguinality becomes the crucial interpersonal orientation, and family of procreation takes precedence over that of orientation. The cost of our increased freedom in marriage choice and domestic privacy is the relative loosening of responsibility toward elders, which may also be seen as a kind of freedom for them, also, provided alternative sources of support are made available.

In the economic sphere, those in occupations which can be handed down from parent to child form an ever smaller proportion of the labor force. Not only does this undermine power over offspring, but also job security in old age. In an employee society, both generations are subject to hiring, firing, and retirement policies over which they have little control. As skill requirements are upgraded, those with more recent training are often able to replace the older, less skilled or at least enter the economy at higher levels. And, as some predict, since human labor becomes a surplus commodity in advanced economies, later entry and earlier exit from production roles will shorten the work lives of individuals, generating large numbers of retired persons regardless of capacities for employment or means of survival. Thus the older person loses whatever resources he or she could command by having the valued

Table A. Level of Analysis

Institutional sphere	Cultural Norms	Social System Statuses	Individual Roles
Economy	Age of retirement Work ethic Valuation of leisure	Worker Retiree Consumer	Socialization to appropriate behavior for these statuses
Polity	Retirement more flexible	Politician, judge, etc.	No socialization problem
	Voting	Voter	Information and access to polls
	Current denigration of age-based experience[1]		
Education	Age-appropriate definition of "student"	Teacher	Socialization for reentry of older students
	Current emphasis on degrees and technical competence	Student	Facilities for older students
	Tenure and mandatory retirement	Retired teacher	Part-time work roles for emeriti
Family	Intergenerational bonds and exchange	Parent Grandparent	Sex and age differences in role availability
	Independence in residence	Widow/widower	Socialization to widowhood
	"Closeness at a distance"	Sibling	Supports from family, services to kin
Religion	Age seen as positive factor, or at least no bar to participation	Clergy Worshiper Social service club member	Socialization and facilities are built into the institution
Health/Welfare	Entitlements to minimal standard of care	Patient Client Provider of services (e.g., RSVP)	Socialization to dependency Facilities and support systems for role playing

[1]Note progressively lower ages of members of Congress and state legislatures.

status of worker, of controlling one's own employment, and of earning an income.

With respect to education, the rapid rate of social change in modern societies and attendant obsolescence of knowledge and skills place the older person at a disadvantage vis-à-vis the more recently educated. Within the family, again, this may make it increasingly difficult to maintain intergenerational authority: Children frequently know more than their parents and are less inclined to accept arbitrary authority. That is, Papa may not know better. In the world at large, cognitive skills frequently serve as a buffer against powerlessness, and some contemporary sociologists go so far as to claim that knowledge will be the future currency of power—those who know, control. While this formulation would appear to place all but the most recently trained at a disadvantage, its effects may be mitigated by a most exciting new concept in education: the possibility of lifelong involvement in learning. Urban universities, community colleges, and all but the most isolated residential post-secondary facilities are not only capable of accepting older students, but may find it economically essential to do so. In the future adult males will find it necessary to retrain or to catch up on the latest advances in their fields, as many do now at the urging of employers or their own best interest. Married women, influenced by the movement toward equality, or having launched their two and one-half children, are returning to college in large numbers—for fun and eventual profit. And some young people, finding all those classroom years too limited, are experimenting with years off to work or gain experience in the world before resuming education. What this suggests for the future is a lifelong blend of work, leisure, and schooling; and for our thesis here today, a lessening of the educational disadvantages of the older person, as well as increased contacts between all age groups in the classroom.

The remaining two spheres—the political and religious areas of activity—have been least affected by the currents noted above, and are in many ways havens of gerontocracy. Years in political service are associated with cumulative power, but even here we can discern some crumbling of prerogatives: The seniority system in Congress, for example, is being challenged; voters are looking for "new faces" and presumably younger ones, as witness the last election which dramatically lowered the average age of Representatives. As for the church, one suspects that an institution whose very purpose is continuity through time, whose aspect is eternal, would be least likely to deny the value of age itself or to hanker after the new, although religious authorities may be challenged by today's generalized questioning of all traditional establishments. Politics and religion are also activities in which the participation of old people is notable: Older citizens have higher voting rates than young adults in the U.S., and older persons are more likely than younger ones to consider religion important in their lives.

Or, using Table B to illustrate the importance of history on the biography of age group members, we need only follow the fate of the aged as societies move from preindustrial modes of subsistence to modern industrial economies. Throughout much of human history, and in all but the most impoverished environments, elders have enjoyed high levels of power, prestige, and material resources, largely through their control over junior members of the family. The disposition of property and marriage partners lay in the hands of

Table B.   Institutional Spheres and Historical Shifts

	Traditional	Modern Industrial
Economy	Owner of land or business which can be handed on to heirs	Employee, subject to mandatory retirement and pensions
	Experience more valuable than technical competence	Unable to pass along occupational status
	Social class placement ascribed	Recent knowledge and skills more marketable than experience
	No set age retirement	
Education	Little required	Increasingly longer periods of training expected
	Elderly as walking encyclopedias	Obsolescence of knowledge
Family	Control over mate selection	Free mate selection
	Strong kinship obligation	Family obligations attenuated—more voluntary than not
	Control over inheritance	
	Family as public institution	Privatized family life
	Call on kin for aid, help	Norm of generational independence
		Other institutions available for aid, service, etc.
Polity	Power accrues with age and control over alliances	Achievement-oriented, universalistic norms of political competence
Religion	Age confers authority, both from experience and nearness to the next world	Religion still seen as refuge for aged, and an area in which they may excel
Health/Welfare	Average life expectancy of four decades	Life expectancies of seven decades, with increasing advantages to women (though greater probability of long widowhood)
	Dependent upon reciprocity of kin	Public provision for income and health care

fathers and uncles, placement in the social order followed from family position. Cultural exhortations to filial piety and the rule of reciprocity protected the parents in their old age. Given typical life expectancies, however, it is unlikely that young adults would have to care for aged parents for any length of time. In preliterate societies, furthermore, the eldest members had the additional advantage of being walking repositories of knowledge. In other cultures, closeness to the gods, whom they would soon join, enhanced the stature of old people. And throughout history, patriarchal religions have both reflected and reinforced the authority of fathers and uncles within families. Although Marxists would claim that control over the means of production—land, weapons, brides, hunting rights—gave older males privileged positions in other institutions, it could as well be argued that their position as head of the family was the grounds for assuming control over all resources, especially since kinship is the organizing principle of most simple societies. Another view would emphasize the psychological orientation toward authoritarianism engendered by patriarchal ideologies, undergirding male dominance in all aspects of life. Whatever the causal chain, the interdependency of social forces is clear, and equally evident is the erosion of every one of these sources of support for the aged under conditions of modern industrialism.

Once this type of overview is presented, the focus can easily shift to contemporary America. My predeliction is to begin with a statistical base; and the Bureau of the Census is very obliging in this respect, having issued special reports in both 1973 and 1976. The demographic profile—numbers, residence, death rates, health status, employment, education, income, life expectancy—is the essential starting point. From there one may wish to shift to the ethnographic approach; that is, the study of old people in a variety of settings going about their daily business in both those social locations which are problematic and problem-producing and those which are conducive to independence and well-being. We often overlook the fact that the great majority of older Americans are doing very well in the face of all sorts of decrements and disabilities. Unfortunately, in some way most of us in the field of gerontology are profiting from the difficulties which beset many elderly, and our focus, accordingly, is on the alleviation or treatment of problems. Nursing homes and geriatric care centers occupy much of our literature, while knowledge of the governmental apparatus and grant-awarding agencies has become a subspecialty. Community-based studies are, however, increasingly common—but these are not easy to fund, and respondents are not always forthcoming. Nonetheless, there is now a research literature on almost any aspect of aging worth studying, and I suspect the next major task for gerontologists will be a grand synthesis of it all. Fortunately, our task is to try to give students the broadest possible perspective on growing old, without necessarily worrying about what it all means—yet.

From the major model (my students call it Hess's all-purpose paradigm) and from the detailed analysis—both census type and ethnographic—of aging in America today, I suspect that enough insight can be garnered to deal with most important topics from the standpoint of our students: What portends for their old age? Have we and they been able to isolate variables and factors conducive to "successful" aging? Are there trends in the broader social system, either inevitable or induced, which will reduce the impediments and enhance the possibilities for long and happy lives?

This last point raises a question which perhaps ought to have been made explicit at the beginning of the course: To what extent can the situation of old people be isolated from that of other age groups? For one thing, the older person has already been a member of other age groups at other historical moments, and these past experiences are what give meaning to the present. If the rate of social change has been such as to render such experiences incomparable to those of persons currently in the younger age groups, there is not much that easily can be shared or learned between generations. Regardless, if where we are is a function of where we've been, then knowing how the generational differences have been shaped will be of some predictive value. But, most important, the old and young coexist, so that we must know how the age groups relate within the several insitutional spheres, for example, or how the same exogenous event may impact differentially on age groups. One attempt to deal systematically with such considerations is the Theory of Age Stratification developed by Matilda White Riley et al. (I'm the second al. from the left.) This perspective treats age groups as strata in much the same way social classes are analyzed. We wish to know the number and composition and other characteristics of each stratum, the nature of interstrata exchanges, and the conditions of intrastratum solidarity or consciousness, etc. One can trace the life course of a given age group, or cut into the ongoing flow of cohorts at one moment in time—the familiar longitudinal and cross-sectional designs—or one might construct a series of life course profiles out of several cross-sectional studies—which we call cohort analysis. What we are looking for ideally is to compare different age cohorts across time; that is, where comparable data exist, to be able to look at what happened, say, to 20 -30 - year–olds in 1900, 1920, 1940, and so on for each designated age cohort. In this fashion we can disentangle recurring idiosyncratic cohort behaviors, have some clue as to what historical events might account for differences in cohort experiences, and tease out whatever constants could then represent pure aging effects.

Cohort analysis may be a bit difficult for undergraduate students, although all that is required is a time series of similar tables, such as successive Gallup polls asking the same question of different aged respondents over several decades. Epidemiological data, when available, are excellent for this purpose; and, with some imagination, much census material is cohortable. However, one suspects that student research projects will of necessity be much more modest—my thinking here is that the course projects could also be used to illustrate the basic techniques of sociological data gathering: Some students may have access to observational niches of interest, others may wish to design and conduct a survey, and still others find happiness in secondary analysis of already published data, even to arranging these in cohort form. If your classes are small enough, you could set aside the last few weeks of class for the students to present informal reports on their findings—I've always found this to be stimulating for the whole class, and one must, often regretfully, cut off debate on what the findings mean.

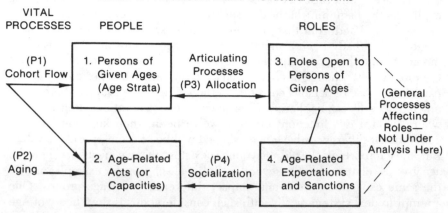

Exhibit 1. Processes Related to Structural Elements

Note: Adapted from *Aging and Society, Volume III: A Sociology of Age Stratification*, M.W. Riley, M. Johnson, and A. Foner (New York: Russell Sage Foundation, 1972). © 1972 by Russell Sage Foundation. Reprinted by permission.

The paradigm for a sociology of age stratification is presented in Exhibit 1. Here the emphasis is upon such structural elements as the number and type of people in a given stratum, and the capacities or behaviors which characterize persons born at particular times, on the one hand; and, on the other, the number and type of roles available to these individuals along with the age-related facilities, sanctions, and normative expectations for role incumbency. Linking the two structural elements are a pair of articulating processes: mechanisms of allocation to roles and socialization to appropriate role behaviors. Cohort flow, then, relates to the movement of persons into roles via selection/allocation processes. Aging can be operationally defined as the temporal changes in capacities, skills, motivations, and so forth which occur within a given cohort. One very simple illustration of the utility of the model would be to examine the experience of persons born during the Great Depression, for instance, as they move through the role structure. This was a very small cohort which reached adulthood as the role system was expanding, which suggests that upward mobility was almost structurally assured. At the other extreme, persons born during the baby boom of 1945–57 will provide a pool of role players possibly in excess of societal capacity, creating a different set of system strains (with personal consequences) especially when they move into their old age. If fertility remains low for another decade, it is quite possible that older people will make up almost one fifth of the American population in 2030. My colleague Joan Waring describes these conditions as the outcome of "disordered cohort flow."

Not only do cohorts flow quantitatively in an orderly and disorderly fashion, but changes take place within societies to affect the quality of cohorts as well. Health status, educational attainment, and adequate socialization facilities all distinguish the capacities of one cohort from another. For example, recent cohort-based research strongly suggests that the presumed declines in intelligence with age may more easily be explained by years of schooling, experience with certain kinds of tests, and test anxiety due to expectations of failure. Some skills improve with age, others may decline, but global measures fail to take these differences into account.

A full explication of the model, along with a number of essays applying it to such diverse topics as science, life course of individuals, friendship, and higher education, may be found in *Aging and Society*, Vol. 3, and in some of the papers collected in *American Behavioral Scientist*, Vol. 19, No. 2 (Nov.–Dec. 1975), edited by Anne Foner. With respect to textbooks in general, there are now a number of inexpensive introductory texts and readers—I think everyone on this panel has written one—so there is no dearth of suitable material. If the college library has the Gerontological Society publications, and *Journal of Marriage and the Family*, and *Social Problems*, there is undoubtedly sufficient resource material for a course in the Sociology of Age. I still feel that doing is learning and have found the field work and research that the students do as a full-term project, with the opportunity to report back to their peers, is a most effective way of promoting gut understanding, the kind of *verstehen* which may be of value to them 50 years or so up the pike.

References

Foner, A. (Ed.). *American Behavioral Scientist*, 1975, *19*, No. 2.

Riley, M. W., Johnson, M., and Foner, A. *Aging and society, volume III: A sociology of age stratification*. New York: Russell Sage Foundation, 1972.

Gerontology in Allied Health Education

Ann Hudis
William Paterson College of New Jersey

In reviewing Betsy Sprouse's excellent tome on educational programs in gerontology (1976), which contains information on gerontological activities of 1,275 colleges and universities in the United States, it was surprising to note that there was no subject heading for "Allied Health" in the index. Attention was given to all the deliverers of health and health-related services, but it would appear that not one school of allied health, of which there are over 1,000 in the United States, offered a course, program, or expressed interest in the area of gerontology, where the needs of the older person would be brought to the attention of all the disciplines working together as a health and social welfare team. It is even more surprising when one considers the fact that there is a growing body of knowledge which supports the concept of gerontology as a prefix or suffix and not a discipline in and of itself.

Allied health education is a complicated set of circumstances. It involves over 16 disciplines, each with its own set of principles, learning experiences, and for many of them, accreditation and/or certification procedures. The term "allied health," when broadly used, includes those personnel who support the work of physicians, dentists, and registered nurses in the areas of patient care, public health, health research, and environmental health. Such persons function at professional, technical, or supportive levels to complement and supplement the activities of the principal health professionals.

An allied health educational program is a planned series of courses at a particular academic level which includes formal classroom instruction, laboratory instruction, and/or clinical training leading to competency in a specific allied health profession or occupation. At the present time, there are approximately 2,300 allied health programs being offered in 719 senior colleges. This does not include allied health programs offered at two-year junior and community colleges.

At the beginning of the twentieth century, there were four recognized health professions: medicine, dentistry, pharmacy, and nursing. Today, over 250 health-related occupations can be identified. It is interesting to note that allied health as a concept is relatively new. It is only since the Second World War that institutions of higher learning have offered academic programs in health and health-related areas in a single department or in an affiliated school or institute. Thus, students representing several disciplines are offered the opportunity to interchange during core and elective courses.

It appears that education and training in allied health began to mature about the same time that interest developed in gerontology. Not only did both areas of interest arrive on the scene about the same time, but both areas represent a multidisciplinary approach to meeting the needs of people. To quote Beattie (1970):

Like Topsy, the field of gerontology has simply grown. Although a few individuals pioneered early efforts in basic research and the provision of specialized services to the aging, gerontology could not be dignified as an area of "organized" concern, whether scientific or applied, until the mid-1940's. However, even at that time early organizational efforts toward the development of a professional and scientific base for gerontology, such as the founding of the Gerontological Society, recognized that gerontology was essentially a part of many disciplines; that is, that it must be approached on a multidisciplinary basis, and indeed, research as well as practice must be envisioned as an interdisciplinary effort.

Every United States President, within recent memory, has made health care concerns a national goal. There is a growing demand for health services due to population growth, rising incomes, better education, expanded health insurance coverage, and governmental financing of health care for the disadvantaged as well as for the aging. All of these factors combine to extract a larger proportion of the national gross product to pay for health services.

All demographic projections indicate that there will be more than 30 million persons over 65 by the year 2000 and that the proportions of older people in the population will continue to increase more rapidly than any other age group in the United States. As soon as there is a major breakthrough in the prevention and treatment of cancer and heart disease, there will be even more people living longer and healthier lives. The emphasis then will be not so much on treatment, but rather on prevention of illness and disease and the promotion and maintenance of good health. Thus, in the immediate and near decades there will be an increasing demand on health and health-related services for older persons.

Current information is that the field of allied health professions is one of the most innovative and rapidly growing of all the health care fields. The schools of allied health are being called upon to educate and to train personnel for increasingly complex services. There is a critical need to ensure that educational progress and career options are designed to enable them to meet the dramatic changes that are occuring in our society. There is no doubt that allied health educators are faced not only with the problem of remaining responsive to changing societal needs but also with severe financial restraints to meet this ever-growing demand.

The organization of health manpower resembles a triangle. At the top, representing approximately one of every eight workers are approximately 500,000 highly trained and educated personnel: physicians, osteopaths, dentists, podiatrists, and optometrists, who have primary responsibility for patient care. The middle level contains almost twice as many personnel: the highly trained allied health workers, such as registered nurses, hospital administrators, medical technologists, physical therapists, health educators, and dietitians, whose education typically ranges from the baccalaureate to the doctorate degree. At the base of the triangle are approximately two million persons who account for five of every eight health care workers and are employed also in allied health occupations that require considerably less education and training than their middle level counterparts.

Despite the rapid growth in employment, manpower in many health care occupations has fallen short of actual demand and need. Shortages of dentists and physicians along with registered nurses are well publicized and have resulted in remedial federal legislation. Shortages in other health occupations are just as serious but less publicized. Also, increased technology and advances in science have led to the development of new occupations such as inhalation therapists and cardiopulmonary resuscitation technicians. Still other programs in allied health have developed to improve the utilization of highly skilled health personnel such as physicians, dentists, and registered nurses by employing workers with less extensive training to perform specified tasks under supervision. Third party payers are just now recognizing the importance of health education as the first level of public health for prevention of illness and disease and the promotion and maintenance of good health.

Needless to say, aging is a dynamic process, constantly buffeted by numerous internal and external factors. Planning, developing, and implementing health programs and services for older persons requires an interdisciplinary approach with a multidisciplinary base of knowledge and skills. A course or program in gerontology is especially needed at the junior college or baccalaureate level because it is at this stage of educational development that the health specialist is being trained to be a practitioner at the "hands-on" level and should be made aware of the special needs of the older person. It is a challenging responsibility to the planners and leaders in allied health to develop curricula which will not only open lines of communication between professions but, since aging is universal and if it is taught as a developmental process, establish aging as a hub of the wheel from which all of the other health disciplines may radiate.

At the very least, an introductory course in gerontology should be part of the core curriculum for allied health students, for this would serve to provide linkages to connect a variety of disciplines. It is in the core concept of allied health that the individual acquires generic information basic to the health field as well as expertise to develop positive attitudes in order to deliver optimum services.

The allied health professional is usually considered a member of the medical "team." The concept of "team care" is not new in terms of its application to human services; the rapid proliferation of teams into many areas of health care delivery is more pronounced today than ever before. Frequently the structure and functions of these teams are based upon a broad range of unrelated applications and ideopathic definitions. The team concept is excellent but commonality is often lacking at the time of training. And again, it is suggested that this task might be met by providing a core course on gerontology for all students in allied health.

Even though training programs in the health sciences may differ in many ways, there seems to be a wide acceptance of the need for practical experience as an integral part of training in allied health. This provides an opportunity for the student to become aware of the linkages of disciplines in meeting the needs of elderly persons. A fieldwork opportunity permits students to relate and test the validity of classroom theory and concepts to practical experience.

Another avenue that must be considered in discussing gerontology as an integral part of allied health education is the career ladder. Many persons in schools of allied health are in "pre-" programs. This is an ideal time to introduce gerontology, not only to create an awareness of their own aging processes, but also to stimulate their interest so as to consider an aspect of gerontology as a career option.

To summarize, the basic idea in developing curricula in gerontology for allied health education is to permit the student to remain within his/her area of specialization while at the same time be able to:

1. Develop an interest in gerontology
2. Gain knowledge in gerontology
3. Apply theories and concepts in gerontology
4. Establish links with other disciplines
5. Become aware of developments in the field
6. Make appropriate referrals
7. Be able to disseminate information
8. Conduct research and study in gerontology
9. Develop positive attitudes towards one's own aging process
10. Be aware of issues and concerns of the aging in society
11. Create an awareness of the field of aging as a career option

References

Beattie, W. M., Jr. Concepts, knowledge and commitment: The education of a practicing gerontologist. *Gerontologist*, 1970, *10*(4, Part 2), 5–11.

Designing curriculum in a changing society, Part I. Englewood Cliffs, N.J.: Educational Technology Publications, Inc., 1970.

Hudis, A. An introductory course in gerontology, development and evaluation. *Gerontologist*, 1974, *14*, 312–315.

McTernan, D. J., and Hawkins, R. O. *Educating personnel for the allied health professions and services*. St. Louis: C. V. Mosby Co., 1972.

Sprouse, B. M. (Ed.). *National directory of educational programs in gerontology*. Madison: University of Wisconsin Press, 1976.

The Psychology of Aging

Margaret H. Huyck
Illinois Institute of Technology

Prerequisites/Assumptions

The following suggestions are offered with the assumption that students will have had, as a minimum, a basic Introduction to Psychology course, introducing them to the substantive areas within the domain of psychology. It would be desirable for students to have had further courses in research design, experimental, physiological, developmental, social, and/or personality psychology. A basic course in the psychology of aging essentially examines these traditional domains of psychology along a time/age dimension—how do these change during the second half of life? In addition, the course may explore domains which are of particular relevance to the geropsychologist (e.g. death and dying).

Reading suggestions were made on the assumption that most students/instructors prefer to have a few "texts" available, rather than a more comprehensive reading list from scattered primary sources. Sometimes there is nothing comparable in the "text" sources, and I have indicated my preference for library-reserve or xerox readings. Obviously, new materials are being published continuously; these suggestions reflect my assessment of the currently available resources.

Texts/Sources

There is, as far as I know, no textbook which adequately and comprehensively covers the domain legitimately "claimed" by psychologists concerned with aging. However, there are several books which include substantial portions:

APA (C. Eisdorfer and M. P. Lawton, Eds.). *The psychology of adult development and aging.* Published by American Psychological Association, 1200 Seventeenth St. N.W., Washington, D.C. 20036, 1973.

Bischof, L. *Adult psychology.* 2nd ed. New York: Harper & Row, 1976.

Botwinick, J. *Aging and behavior: A comprehensive integration of research findings.* New York: Springer Publishing Co., 1973.

Bromley, D. B. *The psychology of human aging.* 2nd ed. Baltimore: Penguin Books, 1974.

Butler, R., and Lewis, M. *Aging and mental health: Positive psychosocial approaches.* St. Louis: C. V. Mosby, 1973.[1]

Substantive Areas for Readings

A. Geropsychology—defining the territory

APA: Zubin, Foundations of gerontology, pp. 3–10.

Bischoff. Adult psychology, pp. 1–73.

Bromley, The concept of human aging; The history of human aging, pp. 15–66.

B. Methodological issues

Botwinick, Research methods: Operational and conceptual issues in research, pp. 290–314.

Bromley, Emergence of scientific methods, pp. 67–77; Methodological issues in the study of human aging, pp. 330–371.

C. Perception and psychophysiology

APA: Thompson and Marsh, Psychophysiological studies of aging, pp. 112–150. Jarvik and Cohen, A biobehavioral approach to intellectual changes with aging, pp. 220–280.

Botwinick, Biological and environmental factors; Simple rigidity, multidimensional rigidity; Contact with the physical environment; Processing sense information; Slow response to environmental stimulation; pp. 70–180.

Bromley, Biological aspects of human aging, pp. 78–121.

Bischof, The adult body, pp. 74–131.

D. Cognition

APA: Arenberg, Cognition and aging, pp. 74–97. Baltes and Labouvie, Adult development of intellectual performance, pp. 157–219.

Bischof, The performing adult, pp. 132–169.

Botwinick, Intelligence; Problem solving; Learning and performance; Aids and types of learning; Memory theory; Retrieving memory; pp. 181–289.

E. Personality and social behavior

APA: Neugarten, Personality change in late life, pp. 311–338. Bennet and Eckman, Attitudes toward aging, pp. 575–597. Lawton and Nahemow, Ecology and the aging process, pp. 619–674.

Bischof, The adult personality; The social adult; Vocations and avocations; Marital status; Family, pp. 166–307.

Bromley, Social aspects of human aging, pp. 122–151; Personality and adjustment in middle and old age, pp. 230–266; Effects of aging on intellectual, social, and athletic achievement, pp. 211–229; The psychopathology of human aging, pp. 238–329.

Botwinick, Sexuality and sexual relations; Turning inward, pp. 35–69.

Gutman, D. Parenthood: A key to the comparative study of the life cycle. In Datan and Ginsberg (Eds.), *Lifespan developmental psychology: Normative life crises*. Washington, D.C.: Academic Press, 1975, pp. 167–184.

F. Special issues: survival, maintenance, and enhancement

Butler, R. and Lewis, M. *Aging and mental health: Positive psychosocial approaches*. St. Louis: C. V. Mosby, 1973.

APA: Gottesman, Quarterman, and Cohn, Psychosocial treatment of the aged, pp. 378–427.

Lieberman, M. Adaptive processes in late life. In Datan and Ginsberg (Eds.), *Lifespan developmental psychology: Normative life crises*, Washington, D.C.: Academic Press, 1975, pp. 135–160.

Kastenbaum, R. Is death a life crisis? On the confrontation with death in theory and practice. In Datan and Ginsberg (Eds.), *Lifespan developmental psychology: Normative life crises*. Washington, D.C.: Academic Press, 1975, pp. 19–50.

Special Projects

There are, obviously, many projects that students can do to "claim" the material as their own, and to help translate summarized research into reality. Such projects are probably best devised by the instructor to reflect the maturity, experience, vocational interests, and energy of the particular class. I try to combine some interaction with a "real person" in an appropriate field setting with a report which demonstrates the ability to evaluate that interaction in terms of the assigned readings and to prepare a written communication in standard English.

Some of the projects which other instructors have found to be useful include:

1. Life history case study—interview designed to elicit the personal story of the individual, in all its complexity, with a particular aim at understanding the interrelationship of the personal, cultural, and historical

2. Comparitive case studies—focused study of two or more individuals,

eliciting life history data but designed to make comparisons on the basis of age, sex, race, social class, identified pathology, etc.

3. Intergenerational study—interviewing two to four members of the same family in different generations, to examine the influence of family and cohort

4. Experimental research replication—using some "classic" experiments in psychology with an older population, and critically evaluating the results in terms of methodological and substantive issues

5. Application of knowledge to applied profession—e.g., on the basis of understanding differential capacities of older adults, design a recreation center, a course in economics, psychotherapy techniques, a communication system, an assembly line

Note

1. Editors' note: A 1977 edition is now available.

Ethnic and Minority Group Content
for Courses in Aging

Aaron Lipman
University of Miami

Textbooks in social gerontology have proliferated at a gratifying rate over the past few years, yet even a cursory scanning of their contents reveals an overriding emphasis on the dominant majority group of the United States aged and a concomitant dearth of material concerning the minority experience. This situation undoubtedly reflects early research patterns which explored the more readily accessible white, middle- and working-class aged population in the United States first, and only later began to investigate the condition of racial and ethnic minorities. However, the present state of the art of gerontology demands not only that the area of minority aging patterns be further investigated, but that some exigency be accorded its inclusion in texts. and courses that teach the principles and dynamics of aging.

Certainly, the impressive body of knowledge that has been accumulated regarding that social category known as "the aged" has been of extreme importance in bringing attention to the plight of those in need, and has been invaluable in serving as an underpinning for the policy decisions and action programs regarding the aged population in the United States. But as we have gotten more sophisticated in our approach, gerontologists have begun to realize that some of the impressions we ourselves helped to propagate have turned out to be erroneous, or at least misleading.

One of the major reasons for this situation was a tendency to contemplate the aged as if they were a unitary homogeneous group, to proceed as if everyone at a certain chronological age was the same and shared the same problems, attitudes, beliefs, values, and reactions. This problem-oriented unitary approach can be said to have been functional, in that it dramatized the plight of the needy aged, and undoubtedly eventuated in swifter action than might have been the case without that sense of urgency generated by the early researchers and the attendant publicity. However, the corollary was the promulgation of the stereotype that the majority of old people in the United States were lonely, socially isolated, below the poverty level, abandoned by their children and families, alienated, and were being dumped into institutions by their uncaring and unfeeling children.

When we as social scientists began to apply a few other variables besides chronological age, we had a difficult time convincing the public that "although a sizeable percentage of older people suffer from poverty, illness and social isolation, the majority of older people are not poverty stricken, socially isolated, rejected by their children or institutionalized" (Lipman, 1976). While the needy among the aged are more numerous than the needy among the young, they are a numerical minority, albeit an important one, of the total aged cohort.

In the same context, we have become aware that within that numerical minority (and probably overlapping in places with the majority) there is a subgroup of racial and ethnic minority aged population clusters that must be clearly delineated, effectively researched, and the results disseminated in texts and lectures that teach social gerontology. The four major minority groups that have been distinguished in the United States, and which should be included in the initial thrust, are the American Indian or native Americans, black Americans, Asian Americans, and Spanish-speaking Americans.

In studying the minority aged, we need to collect a body of knowledge which will indicate uniformities in the minority experience of aging, as contrasted with the dominant group, as well as showing the effects of subcultural differences between various minorities.

Yet in our effort to derive meaningful theoretical generalizations as well as workable policies and action programs for the minority aged, we must again avoid the error of implicit social, psychological, and valuational homogeneity. While there are undoubtedly certain correlates to poverty and minority living, there is little question that the native American experience differs from that of the black, which differs from that of the Puerto Rican, which differs from that of the Japanese.

For example, in gerontological literature, it is a datum that the elderly population is predominantly female. While this is true for the Japanese American, Kalish has indicated that the Chinese American elderly population is predominantly male. Presumably, the explanation for this lies in the fact that while the Japanese emigrated to the United States in families, the Chinese population that emigrated to the United States consisted mainly of unaccompanied males. What will comparable data yield for ensuing generations (Kalish and Moriwaki, 1973)?

That fund of knowledge we already possess concerning the minority elderly indicates that as a group, they are more economically disadvantaged than those elderly that belong to the dominant group. Yet while attention has been given to social class differences, research has neglected to account for variations within or across class lines due to the interplay of racial or ethnic factors. Part of the problem with data concerning the poor is the confounding of the concepts "poor" and "minority." For the total population at all ages, the likelihood of being poor if one is a member of a minority is four times as great as for that of the dominant group. By the time a person reaches old age, that proportion is down to twice as great (Butler, 1973). This is not necessarily due to an improvement in the fortunes of the poor elderly minority member as he gets old, but more probably to the fact that so small a number survive to old age. In 1975, the median income for white families was $14,268, compared with $9,551 for Hispanics and $8,779 for black families. "Nearly 27 percent of Hispanics were below the federally defined poverty level of $5,500 for an urban family of four, compared with 9.7 percent of whites and 31.3 percent of blacks" (New York Times, 1976). In 1975, for those 65 years and over, 13.4 percent of the whites were below the poverty level compared with 32.7 percent of the Hispanics and 36.3 percent of the blacks.

When one realizes that an older person has been a minority group member for a much longer time than he has been (or ever will be) an aged person, it becomes evident that membership in a minority group supersedes and probably has greater salience for the individual than membership in an elderly aged cohort. How he will age, his perceptions of his aged status and situation, and the type of action he will take to manipulate his environment will, to a great extent, be functions of belonging to this minority group. Furthermore, the very core question of whether he will survive his environment long enough to become old in our society appears to be closely correlated with the fact of his minority status. Thus, we find that while blacks constitute 11 percent of the general population, they constitute only 7.8 percent of the elderly.

In terms of life expectancy, American Indians or native Americans live 44 years; for Mexican Americans it is estimated at 57 years (Butler, 1973)—at a period when the "total population" has an estimated life expectancy of 72.4 (HEW, 1976). This means that for a very sizeable number of Americans in the above categories, neither Social Security nor Medicare will ever influence their lives in any way, since they will not live long enough to collect benefits from these programs. If we exclude infant mortality, the average age of those dying in 1962–67 was 53 years for native Americans and 59½ years of age for nonwhites, as compared to 68½ years for whites (Special Committee on Aging, 1973).

Racial minority members have high visibility and are easily identifiable. As a consequence of individual and institutional racism, they have suffered the cumulative effects of prejudice, subordination, negative stereotyping, discrimination, economic deprivation and exploitation, and general degradation and humiliation. There is also a disproportionate victimization of the minority individual in terms of predatory crimes and violence, on the one hand, and linked with a prejudicial criminal justice system on the other.

For the minority persons who do grow old in a hostile and exclusionary larger society, there has been a cumulative input of all the above influences which, as we know from the dynamics of human behavior, must have had a significant impact on the aging process for those individuals. Furthermore, in addition to those mentioned above, they now have the added strain of agism with which to contend. This is the phenomenon referred to as the "multiple jeopardy" of the minority aged, in facing the combined assaults of racism, agism, and poverty.

Statistically, we know that these minority group members are likely to have the least supply of those resources which are important in successfully coping with the aging process—such resources as income, health, educational level, and social participation (Lipman, 1966). There is also evidence that despite their greater need, they underutilize the many and diverse special services that have been provided for the aged population in recent years.

Frances Carp (1970) found, for example, that in one community, although Mexican Americans constituted about half the population, "and an even larger proportion of persons eligible for public housing," only 3 percent of the Mexican Americans applied for public housing for the elderly. Ninety-seven percent of the applicants were Anglo-Americans, although they made up only 40 percent of the population. Even conscious efforts to maximize the number of Mexican Americans for the next facility (which was built nine years later) resulted in only a slight increase in applicants with Spanish surnames. How do we accommodate to or change these patterns of behavior in order to make our institutional supports available to the minority elderly?

In the attempt to reach these group members with available services, we must first ascertain whether the services are adequate or appropriate for their needs, or whether new, specially designed programs will have to be instituted. If the programs are appropriate and needy people are still not utilizing them, does the fault lie with the means of publicizing these programs? Are the proper channels of communication being employed to reach the groups for whom the programs were designed? If these people are aware of the programs and still do not avail themselves of the services, is there some cultural barrier that is preventing them from doing so? Is it a characteristic of that group that they will not initiate action, or have no skill in manipulating their environment, or cannot or will not cope with bureaucratic constraints?

In accord with the foregoing discussion, it can be seen that it is important to include material about minority groups in our curricula on aging for a number of reasons: There is the purely epistemological aim of scientifically expanding our theoretical generalizable base of knowledge concerning the total gerontic population. Secondly, comparative studies on the adjustment of different groups to aging could identify the dynamics that contribute to that adjustment; and by identifying those coping structures and mechanisms which work for variant subcultural groups in our society, we might also refine our knowledge of the dominant group adaptation process. Finally, knowledge about minority groups would help generate action programs and policies targeted for those individuals who, as a consequence of their membership in an ethnic or racial minority subgroup, have not been reached by programs which were designed by and for the dominant white majority.

References

Butler, R. N. *Why survive? Being old in America*. New York: Harper & Row, 1973, 6.

Carp, F. Communicating with elderly Mexican-Americans. *Gerontologist*, 1970, 9, 126–134.

HEW, Monthly Vital Statistics Report, Provisional Statistics, Annual Summary for the United States, 1975. (HRA) 76–1120, 24(13), June 30, 1976.

Kalish, R. A., and Moriwaki, S. The world of the elderly Asian American. *Journal of Social Issues, 1973, 29* (2).

Lipman, A. Resource utilization in community support systems. In William C. Martin and Albert J. E. Wilson III (Eds.), *Aging and total health*. Eckerd College Gerontology Center, 1976, pp. 109–120.

Lipman, A. Responsibility and morale. *Proceedings of the Seventh Congress International Association of Gerontology* (Vienna, 1966). Wien, Med, Akad, Vienna, 1966, 267–276.

Harris, Louis, et al. *The myth and reality of aging in America, A study for the National Council on Aging*. Washington, D.C.: 1975.

Special Committee on Aging, United States Senate. *Advisory Council on the Elderly American Indian*. Washington, D.C.: U.S. Government Printing Office, 1973, 13.

Gerontology and Geriatrics in Professional Curricula of Medical Schools

J. Paul Sauvageot[1]
The University of Akron

Just as gerontology is the science of aging, geriatrics is the application of medical science in the health care of the elderly.

We know that the primary causes and courses of aging are gene coded or genetic, are multifaceted, and are sealed at the time of conception. They are species and individually specific and determine possibilities for average and maximal life spans.

The secondary causes of aging are environmental—internal and external—and operate from conception throughout life. Included in the secondary factors are such entities as nutrition, trauma, acute and chronic diseases, intoxications, intelligence, life style, habits, and socioeconomic and ecological factors, plus luck.

The interactions of primary and secondary causes determine the pattern of total and regional aging at any time. There is no fixed ratio between age in years and the manifestations of aging.

Geriatrics is that subspecialty of medicine which applies the science and art of medicine and surgery to the diseases, organ deficiencies, and deformities encountered in elderly persons, particularly in those 65 years of age and older.

Although geriatrics lies at the opposite end of the rainbow from pediatrics, I assure you that it is just as important technically, humanistically, and socioeconomically to patients between 65 and 100 years as pediatrics is to patients from in-utero to adolescence.

It should be apparent to medical educators that one cannot teach geriatrics to undergraduate medical students without first teaching the fundamentals of the forerunner and sister science of gerontology.

To put it another way, a skilled gerontologist without being a physician, can accomplish great things for his or her science and for the welfare, life style, and happiness of the elderly. However, to be a skilled geriatrician one must be a good gerontologist and practice the skills of each discipline in treating patients.

There are some 23 million Americans—around 11 percent of the population—in all strata of society who desperately need the services of current knowledge in gerontology and geriatrics. Fortunately they are getting rapidly increasing help from the mushrooming higher educational gerontology programs in colleges and universities around the country, particularly from applied gerontology in hundreds of programs at all levels of government and private sectors.

However, I am sorry and ashamed to tell you that geriatrics is a large and almost neglected area of the practice and study of primary general internal medicine.

The first of this month I talked with Mr. Herman Gruber of the AMA Department of Education. He told me that in 1976 of 112 accredited schools granting M.D. degrees, not one had mandatory or required curriculum in either gerontology or geriatrics. However, 45 of them offer electives in geriatrics but not in gerontology. Mr. Gruber does not know at what level of training the electives are offered. He does not have available data on the number of students involved, in which schools, nor the length and content of the electives. The courses are offered in the departments of primary care, community medicine, and internal medicine.

Mr. Gruber said that he personally has been pushing at AMA headquarters for starting this long neglected field of study at premedical and medical school levels. I learned further that Dr. Leonard D. Fenninger, AMA Group Vice President for Medical Education, will meet next month with representatives of the American Association of Medical Colleges, the American Geriatric Society, and the American Gerontological Association. The purpose is to talk seriously about introducing gerontology and geriatrics into required medical school curricula.

I cannot help but feel there may be new geriatric and gerontological courses now offered—and stressed—at a few medical schools, especially those in proximity to outstanding gerontology centers—north, east, south, and west. Perhaps such courses have been initiated since the 1976 data were accumulated.

All of us are aware that the elderly require considerably more care than the other 89 percent of the population. Consider, too, that the annual average health bill for individuals 65 and over is two and one half times that for persons between 19 and 64 and six times that for youth.

Why, then, the unprecedented gap in medical teaching? Here are some of the reasons:

1. Our youth-oriented society
2. The dogmatism of medical schools against change
3. Medical prejudices against elderly patients with chronic diseases as being uninteresting, with cost ineffectiveness in therapeutic effort
4. Today's spotlight on acute cures and spectacular results
5. The medical schools' political and economic advantages for short- and long-term basic and clinical research with the "paper mill" necessity of frequently published papers on progress and results
6. The gerontologically ridiculous compulsory retirement age of 65 plus the American worship of the gross national product
7. The real paucity of dedicated, knowledgeable, trained geriatricians in medical schools, hospitals, and among practicing physicians

Now—what are the forces reaching ground swell proportions in recent years causing a turnabout in medical curricular thinking? Here are a few:

1. The stark number of the elderly with increasing proportionality throughout the rest of this century
2. The accruing effects of the Older Americans Act and the Administration on Aging of the federal government in the 1960s—together with the 1971 White House Conference on aging
3. The work of state commissions on aging in all 50 states
4. The wide dissemination of gerontological knowledge
5. Service and educational programs for the elderly throughout most large municipalities and counties in the nation
6. The increasing political clout of the organized elderly through such organizations as AARP, NRTA, and other groups
7. The ascendency of the importance of the primary care physician in the health care system and hence in medical schools

The recently established Northeastern Ohio Universities College of Medicine, commonly called NEOUCOM, has an entirely new concept in medical education. It comprises a consortium of three geographically close state universities—The University of Akron, Kent State, and Youngstown State University combined with the new medical school. The six-year, 24-quarter program confers both B.S. degrees and M.D. degrees and utilizes teaching community hospitals in three cities for hospital, clerkship, and postgraduate education.

Through the influence of a committee of Akron-based Area Agency on Aging 10B we were able to readily get a commitment from NEOUCOM to teach gerontology and geriatrics.

The road ahead will be difficult for some years because of lack of faculty with expertise and because of budgetary constraints. But we must move ahead.

Existing geriatric experts will have to be utilized in teaching in many medical schools through the use of movies, TV, tapes, and self-instructional computers for both didactic and clinical demonstration purposes. It seems to me that the same techniques must be used to teach gerontology and geriatrics to hospital-based physicians and house staff and as credit courses for other physicians.

Medical schools will advise or require that certain minimal courses in gerontology be taken in premedical college training and as a prerequisite for medical school admission.

May we all rejoice in the turnaround that is imminent, but strive even harder to enhance the progress.

Note

1. Editors' note: We are sad to announce the death of the distinguished physician, Jean Paul Sauvageot, on October 21, 1977.

Gerontology in Professional and Preprofessional Curricula

Bernita M. Steffl
Arizona State University

Introduction

Even though older individuals have always occupied the greatest percentage of hospital beds and are the biggest consumer of health services, we have not planned to meet the special needs of this group with any reasonable degree of special preparation. For example, textbooks used for human development courses until recently ended at early adulthood. We would not think of sending a nurse or teacher to work with children without some knowledge about behaviors and feelings of children, but we have not prepared so well for our work with the elderly.

As far back as 1968 it was pointed out that the advent of Medicare would bring us (nursing educators) face to face with health care needs of the aged and the lack of health professionals and paraprofessionals prepared to respond to the needs.

So where are we in 1977? I like to think that we've come a long way and that, as someone stated at the International Congress on Gerontology in Israel in 1975, "Hopefully we are at the end of the beginning." We now know that much early research described characteristics of groups of aged congregated in poor farms, nursing homes, and state mental hospitals, leading to a general picture of impaired elderly. This created negative stereotypes regarding characteristics of the elderly. It created pity and revulsion and certainly added to the development of negative attitudes toward the aged in our youth-oriented, production-oriented society. We are now busy dispelling those myths and convincing ourselves that most older people are a capable, valuable, self-sustaining, significant, and necessary segment of society and that they do respond to medical treatment, nursing intervention, and social services.

Developing Content

Major ingredients and steps in curriculum development in gerontological nursing are: (1) teachers prepared in gerontology versus geriatrics, (2) theory based on quality research, (3) clinical practice linked with theory, (4) a focus on health versus illness, (5) to include content on prevention, health maintenance, and self-health assessment, and (6) a multidisciplinary approach to research, teaching, and practice for ultimate comprehensive, coordinated continuity of care for the aged.

As stated above, content and experience for nursing education in gerontology needs to be carefully planned by design, based on scientific rationale, and conceptualized into a theoretical framework for teaching and learning. This sounds simple but is very difficult and takes a well prepared and skilled teacher. For example, take the voluminous research theories on memory loss, short-term and long-term memory, and link that to learning process; and try putting it into a simple package so that the practicing nurse or paraprofessional can use the valuable results of this research at the bedside. This is what needs to be done!

In this short period of time I will try only to describe how one begins— how I began—and what has worked for me. I like to use Bloom's Taxonomy as a guide for developing objectives and for determing at what levels to place content. It is helpful in determining prerequisites as well as expected behavioral outcomes. The Continuing Education Department at our College has used this taxonomy in specific guidelines to help faculty develop C.E. content at a variety of levels. For a review of Bloom's Taxonomy see Figure 1. Some of you may not care for this concept. There are other instructional systems and models that may work for you, such as Banathey's Systems Approach and Mager's Behavioral Objectives. We owe it to our students to state student-centered expected behavioral objectives and you are probably as aware as I am of the fact that many college professors do not know how to do this very well.

In nursing, until recent years we tended to follow a medical model and focus on the content of care for the aged was disease and hospital centered. Even now it seems hard for some professionals to envision the patient out of the hospital. We often end up too "geriatric" centered instead of gerontological. There is danger of focusing on senility versus senesence. No one person is all sick or all well at any time. It is much better to look at what is left, not what is gone. I believe our first emphasis should be on understanding the feelings and behaviors of old people, and after that, dealing with the needs, losses, and infirmities is easier and more apt to be successful. This, then, is how I

Figure 1. Guide for Writing Behavorial Objectives and Identifying Levels of Learning

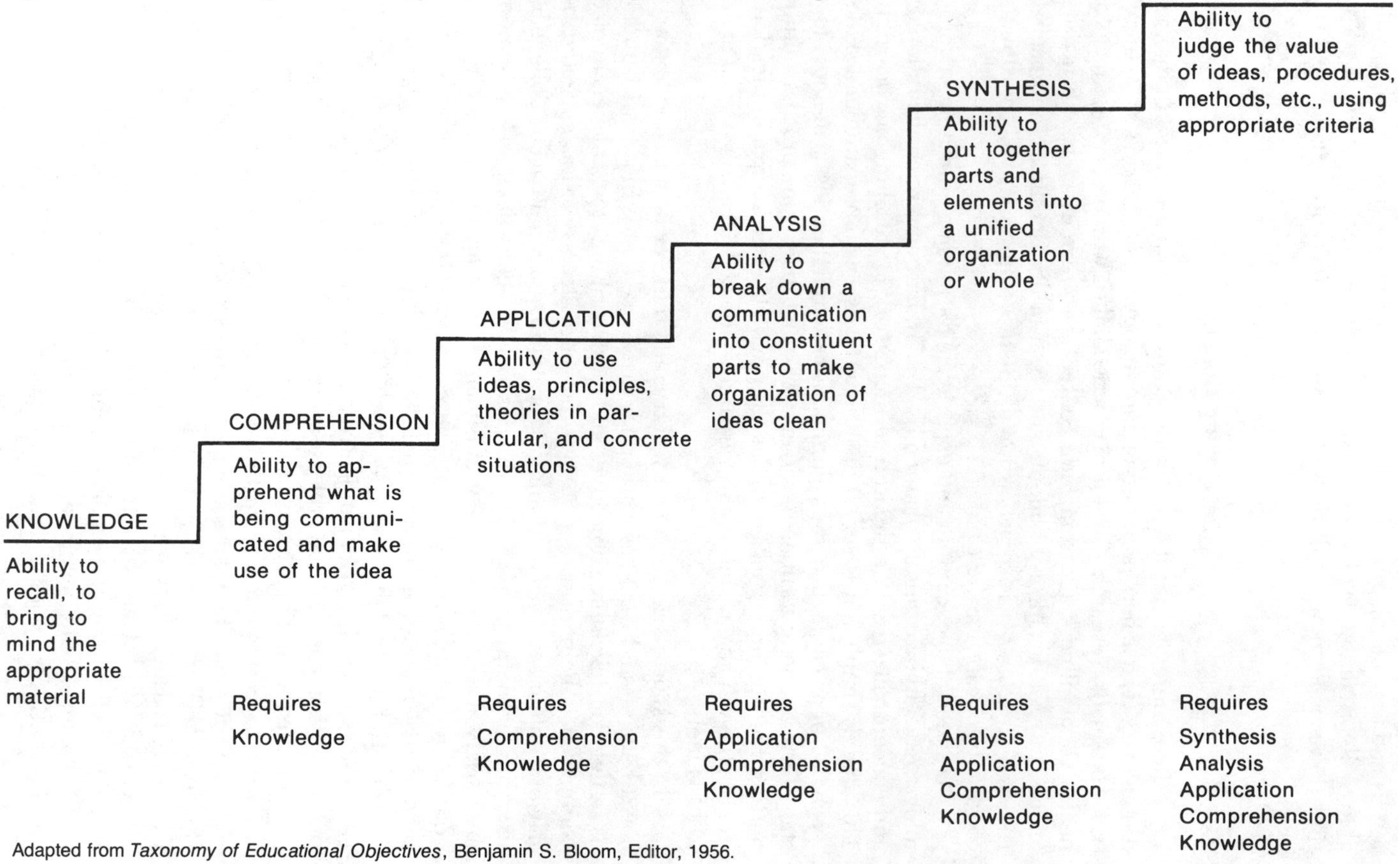

EVALUATION

Ability to judge the value of ideas, procedures, methods, etc., using appropriate criteria

SYNTHESIS

Ability to put together parts and elements into a unified organization or whole

ANALYSIS

Ability to break down a communication into constituent parts to make organization of ideas clean

APPLICATION

Ability to use ideas, principles, theories in particular, and concrete situations

COMPREHENSION

Ability to apprehend what is being communicated and make use of the idea

KNOWLEDGE

Ability to recall, to bring to mind the appropriate material

Requires
Knowledge

Requires
Comprehension
Knowledge

Requires
Application
Comprehension
Knowledge

Requires
Analysis
Application
Comprehension
Knowledge

Requires
Synthesis
Analysis
Application
Comprehension
Knowledge

Adapted from *Taxonomy of Educational Objectives*, Benjamin S. Bloom, Editor, 1956.

start developing basic content (see Figure 2). I use this matrix because aging has biophychosocial components and individuals age in three dimensions. There are norms and theories for each of these components and great individual differences. In fact, the rate of biological, psychological, and sociological aging may be different in the same individual (Woodruff and Birren, 1975).

This model will of course have many more components—smaller modules of specialized content. For this we need a variety of perspectives and the expertise and research findings of multidisciplines. At this point in my thinking, I do not believe gerontology is a distinct discipline. I would be hard pressed to define a generic major—and will be interested in learning more about the program at Molloy College in New York, which does so.

In nursing we draw heavily from other disciplines. A problem we have, though, is in educating the public and other disciplines that professional nursing has a strong generic base in the social and behavioral sciences as well as the natural sciences; that our focus is on health care—not just sick care; that many of our courses would be useful as electives in your programs; and, that you ought to use us more in the multidisciplinary approach. I believe we have a contribution and if I had to pinpoint a specific one I would say in assessment skills.

Concerns and Issues

As important as what we put in the curriculum, and what we teach, is who is doing the teaching? Hudis and others have stated that "Persons selected to

Figure 2.   Curriculum in Gerontology:
The Matrix of Gerontological Content in This Model
Uses "Basic Human Needs" as the Foundation

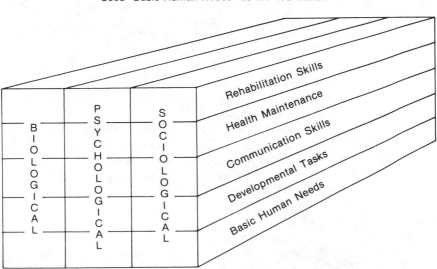

teach a course in gerontology should be trained and skilled not only in education but also in the field of aging" (1974). I believe we must, and perhaps this organization (AGHE) should address itself now to credentialing of teachers in gerontology or developing some guidelines for qualifications of those teaching in the field. With the explosion of interest and funded programs, I'm sorry to say we have people working in and teaching gerontology who are not well prepared in gerontology or teaching. This is a major concern and it is costly in terms of program input and consumer outcomes.

Some of the more specific issues that educators have to struggle with are:

1. Placement of gerontology content in the total curriculum. We are always adding and never taking out, and therefore, sometimes watering down or diluting content to a dangerous point. Some would argue that the students can get much by assigned independent study. I believe that at an under-graduate level independent study needs very well-defined guidelines and guidance and it does not shorten the curriculum. (I speak from five years experience in an integrated curriculum where this was tried.)

2. The issue of graduate-undergraduate content in gerontology is a cru-cial one. As Seltzer has stated since 1974, we need to make some decisions about this. The problem is that most professionals of all levels are just tuning in to gerontology, and the orientation and needs for the graduate student or the practicing professional with an advanced degree are often the same in content as for the undergraduate, but these people insist on graduate level labels, even for continuing education units. In nursing, I believe we have come to some general consensus on this issue; at least exploration with faculty from a number of different university programs indicates that in the undergraduate program the focus of theory and practice for the beginning student is on understanding and communicating with the "well" older adult who is func-tioning in his "normal" or "natural" community setting. In subsequent levels the student learns more about pathophysiology (in old age) and technical intervention skills. In the final level of undergraduate preparation the student should be able to plan and contribute to comprehensive, coordinated con-tinuity of care. Though the undergraduate student needs to be aware of the need for researched information, I believe the major focus for graduate level preparation in gerontology should be on exploring the research and in de-veloping clinical specialization.

3. What kind of clinical experience should we provide and how much? Clinical practice in nursing is not limited to technical and intrusive proce-dures. Any kind of face-to-face or heart-to-heart interaction with old people is valuable clinical experience for the student and it must come before work with the acutely ill patient or rehabilitative intervention skills. In my teaching and in my courses in gerontology I place heavy emphasis on learning to under-stand the feelings and behaviors of old people and developing assessment skills. I believe these are basic to all other skills for working with the aged.

4. Should we prepare nurse specialists in gerontology, practitioners, or geropsychiatric nurse specialists? This is a very pressing question. It is so

pressing that there is real controversy and confusion within the profession as well as in the public about the expanded and extended roles of nursing. The provider agencies have helped confuse us and the consumer suffers. They want us to provide special training for expanded roles in geriatrics but want us to do it within existing undergraduate program curricula. They do not want to pay for specialized training.

I believe that *we do need to provide basic knowledge and skills in gerontological nursing in basic programs*, but I also believe we need specialization and expanded roles to help provide care that the aged are not receiving right now. There need to be specialists and practitioners to bridge the gaps and lack of medical supervision of the infirm elderly, especially in geropsychiatry. A recent government report indicates that the highest incidence of new cases of psychopathology of all types in the United States is found in the population over age 65. A WHO Report states the incidence of mental health problems in those over age 65 is 236 in 100,000 and two and one-half times greater than the rate in the next highest age group. The estimate is that 10–25 percent of elderly in the community have emotional problems, yet fewer than 4 percent of patients seen in public or private mental health centers are over age 65. The suicide rate increases with age. Seventy-five percent of suicides in this country are in the age over 65 group. This is an impressive figure when one realizes this is from only 10 percent of the population.

5. Also a concern is the quality and quantity of research which is available and relevant to the development of curricula for the helping professions. Research in the social sciences is limited. It is more difficult to document than biological and does not get equal preference for funding—at least not on my campus. There is great need for more researched information regarding medication and drugs used by the elderly and the many facets of organic brain syndrome. Both of these involve behaviors and are hard to research.

Continuing Education

Though I am speaking mainly to basic education today a word must be said about the curriculum needs in continuing education for nurses in gerontology (and other helping professionals, for that matter). Current research indicates that we are in an age or point in time where we can no longer obtain our lifetime education in one period of time or at one point in our life. In the future, the average professional may have to update his knowledge and skills as often as three times during his career.

At this time continuing education programs and efforts are just beginning to scratch the surface. This will be another big task for AGHE. In nursing we are very aware of this because all state professional organizations are looking at mandatory continuing education for relicensure. Nine states have passed laws to this effect.

A clear or better distinction needs to be made between workshop and conference content versus regular college courses. This kind of content needs to be evaluated by a curriculum committee to see how it fits with other educational goals. In our Continuing Education Department, all course offerings are evaluated by a committee with representatives from the graduate and undergraduate programs. I believe we need more continuing education via organized courses (even short courses) for credit. I have some questions in regard to the world of workshops. The present smorgasbord is attractive and tasty—but costly and sometimes hard to piece together for the kind of foundations we are trying to build.

Summary

The key ingredients and steps in curriculum development in gerontology include:

+ Teachers prepared in gerontology versus geriatrics
+ A theoretical framework based on research
+ Linking theory to clinical experience
+ Focusing on health versus illness
+ Prevention, health maintenance, and self-health assessment
+ A multidisciplinary approach to research and practice

References

Bloom, B. S., et al. *Taxonomy of educational objectives, the classification of educational goals*. New York: David McKay, 1956.

Elias, M. F., Hickey, T., Spinetta, J., Urban, H., Watson, W., Schai, K. W., Wilson, A., Sinex, J. M., Johnson, F. R., Beattie, W. M., Jr., and Weg, R. B. Symposium: The real world and the ivory tower, etc. *Gerontologist*, *14*(6), 1974, 525–553.

Frenay, A. C., Sr. Helping students work with the aging. *Nursing Outlook*, July 1968, 44–46.

George, J. A. Teaching the young about the old. *Nursing Outlook*, June 1972, 405–407.

Hickey, T. In service training in gerontology. *Gerontologist*, *14*(1), 1974, 57–64.

Hickey, T., Spinetta, J. J., Peterson, D. A., Connelly, J. R., and Weg, R. B., Symposium: Educational intervention and education. *Gerontologist*, *15*(5), 1975, 423–451.

Hudis, A. An introductory course in gerontology. *Gerontologist*, *14*(4), 1974, 312–315.

Moses, D. V., and Lake, C. S., Geriatrics in the baccalaureate nursing curriculum. *Nursing Outlook*, July 1968, 41–43.

Seltzer, M. M. Education in gerontology. *Gerontologist*, *14*(4), 1974, 308–311.

Woodruff, D. S., and Birren, J. E. *Aging: Scientific perspectives and social issues*. New York: The Van Nostrand Company, 1975, 8.

Social Work: Gerontology in Professional and Preprofessional Curricula

Sheldon S. Tobin
University of Chicago

Gerontology in social work curricula refers both to the study of the aging process and to social work practice with the aging. When, for example, we discuss influencing a faculty member to consider the last half of the life span in a course in human behavior or we are ourselves developing a course on adult development and aging, we are focusing on gerontology as a discipline. Our intent, however, is not only to educate students interested in aging in the essential knowledge base, but also to sensitize all students, as well as faculty, to the processes of aging and, in turn, to the aging as an important target group for the entire range of social work interventions. Specific courses on interventions, however, are also essential—including methods courses and field experiences.

Invariably, therefore, a program in gerontology at the undergraduate or the graduate level will include, on the one hand, courses in aging as a developmental process and the older cohort in contemporary society and, on the other hand, social treatment with, or planning and policy formulation for the aged, as well as field experiences with agencies who work directly with the aged or who plan, develop, or implement programs for the aged.

Is this all there is to curriculum development? Fortunately not! Life in the ivory tower would be much too simple for all of us talented educators. Challenging us are such questions as: What is the appropriate quantity of gerontological content in a social work program? To what extent must a viable program include practice approaches as diverse as treatment, integration of services, planning, and policy formulation and implementation? (In the current *lingua franca*: micro, mezzo, and macro intervention.) What does influencing others—in one's own academic unit and in other units because gerontology is "by nature interdisciplinary"—really mean? What level of sophistication and practice expertise do we want, or hope for, in our B.A. and M.A. products? Answers to these questions are a little harder than to the question responded to in my opening remarks on the essentials of a curriculum.

Yet we must try to address the question of how much of the curriculum do we want. My own approach follows the old adage of "minimal intervention." Much, if not most, of my initial efforts in developing a program at the M.A. level for a diverse set of practitioners was to elicit others to add gerontological contents to their courses and to develop field placements related to aging within their own orientation. The gerontology program, consequently, is perceived by the casework faculty; the applied behavioral analysis faculty; the treatment of families, individuals and groups faculty (the tasty FIG program); the community work faculty; the health policy faculty; and, hopefully, by the other faculty groups—as not "messing with their turf." Facilitating the political process in my own case were such "tricks of the trade" as providing training funds to support our shared students, a willingness to teach courses helpful to the variety of faculty clusters, consultation to faculty on curricula as well as personal problems with aging family members, availability to the many students who needed help in writing papers related to gerontology, and assuming responsibility for advising and supervising field placements for students focusing on the area of social planning for the aged. Thus I have attempted to resolve the dilemma of how much gerontology versus how much else by developing fewer courses and more bridges, with an eye on tapping into the expertise of my fellow faculty members.

The second challenging question of the breadth of the program is reflected in my approach to "spreading the gospel," but not entirely. Although I want my students to have a beginning expertise in *all* methods of intervention, it is not possible in any curriculum of reasonable length. I may wish to have my students (at least most of them) for five, or even ten, years instead of two, but I know this is unrealistic. The best I can do within two years is to encourage each student to have a beginning expertise in a more narrowly focused intervention strategy and an exposure to, as well as appreciation for, other strategies. To reduce my discomfort related to this dilemma, I offer a course, titled "Aging: Process and Planning," for students in the various sequences or concentrations where, more through the students' interaction than the formal course content, cross-fertilization occurs. Fortunately the findings of a study of all 1970 graduates, three years after beginning practice, suggest that social workers rather rapidly move from one job to another and from one set of functions to another. It is not uncommon for the student singularly committed to casework to become the budget-juggling administrator, or for the incipient evangelistic policy maker to become the deliverer of direct services—both within a few short years of graduation. To package, therefore, the precise set of practice courses that I feel is warranted or that a student desperately wants may be quite unnecessary. Maybe the most we can do is provide a solid launching pad for a career that may take many turns, but one that (from our data on veterans, graduates of the SSA classes from 1947 to 1952) is invariably very self-fulfilling.

The third question I posed, regarding influencing others, has also been touched on above. But not answered is how to extend social work programs outward to maximize an interdisciplinary approach. I was fortunate because of the existing expertise on campus. Yet I am also confronted with federal guidelines for multidisciplinary centers on aging (that is, if I am greedy enough to want training monies) that may not be congruent with the wishes of the all-campus faculty group. Because this topic is one that will be covered in other discussions, I shall turn to the fourth question.

What do we want from our BSW and MSW products? Here the question is not simply that of curriculum content. Rather the question is of the relationship between undergraduate and graduate education. If the B.A. level social worker is to be the direct practitioner and the M.A. level social worker the planner, the policy analyzer formulates and implements—then not only will our programs by level have to articulate better, but we will also have to shape our programs accordingly. Moreover, a concern of mine is that we shall have to redefine means of effectively bridging the world of academia and practice. For example, I may have to equip my M.A. graduates to become educators themselves, primarily in agencies employing B.A. direct practitioners, but also in undergraduate programs. Indeed the ramifications of the B.A. degree as the first professional degree have hardly been felt at either M.A. or B.A. levels. How we, as social work educators and as educators specifically interested in gerontology, respond is too early to forecast. Because, however, of our mutual interest in gerontology, B.A. and M.A. gerontological educators may be able to make a unique contribution to the current debate.

I have touched on only a few questions related to curriculum. Others exist and are surely to receive attention in other sessions. Questions such as: Are the differences in orientations of schools beneficial for gerontological educators? What is unique to graduates of social work programs? Can we justify institutional and federal funding for our social work training programs?

Yes, we have many challenging questions. Fortunately in the challenge lies excitement and gratification!

A Systems Approach to Program Evaluation

R. O. Washington
The Ohio State University

One of the basic principles of democracy is that public servants and organizations entrusted with the responsibility and authority to use public resources for the well-being of citizens have also the responsibility to render a full accounting of their activities. This form of accountability is ingrained in our governmental process, and is carried over into higher education as well as other fields of human services.

Practitioners in the field of gerontology have come to accept evaluation and other measures of accountability much in the same way as we have other human services workers. We have come to realize that program evaluation is not simply a form of accountability imposed upon service providers by program funders whose major concern is the eradication of waste, duplication, and inefficiency in service delivery; but rather, to respect program evaluation as an essential process in overall decision making.

The idea of program evaluation, as a fundamental, and constitutive element of human services management is relatively new. Historically, human services workers evaluated programs in terms of inputs rather than outcomes. Heretofore, we have relied too heavily upon such indices as staff training and experience, size and amount of budgets, the improvement of sites and facilities rather than on improvement in the life styles and life chances, the physical, social, and emotional well-being or other indices of directed social change among service recipients. While measures of input are essential in assessing program effectiveness, they should not outweigh process or out-come measures, the three of which underlie the logical framework of a systems approach to program evaluation. However, before we link the systems approach to program evaluation, perhaps some discussion of each concept separately is warranted.

The Systems Approach

So-called "systems" thinking became popular in the behavioral sciences a little more than a quarter of a century ago. It was conceived as an alternative to the overworked equilibrium and organismic perspectives of society and the nature of man which had been in vogue for some time. The new boy on the block, created from general systems theory, cybernetics, and information or communication theory,[1] and clothed in the languages of systems analysis, operations research, and management science, called attention to the concept of a whole system. Underlying this concept was the notion that systems are made up of sets of components that work together for the overall objective of the whole. In other words, a whole which functions as a whole by virtue of the interdependence of its parts is called a system, and the method which aims at discovering how this is brought about in the widest variety of systems has been called general systems theory (Buckley, 1968).

One should make clear at the outset, however, that a general systems approach is not the same as the application of systems analysis. Systems analysis is defined here as the application of systematic methods to a task or problem. A systems approach, as already stated, involves beginning with the perspective of the *total system* and working downward through all the subsystems, always staying within the framework and the constraints of the system. This process is generally recognized as a deductive (general to specific, or "top down") method, as compared to the inductive method, more commonly associated with the scientific method.

Using this line of reasoning, then, the systems approach is simply a way of thinking about these total systems and their components. It concerns itself above all with the nature of decision making, and has a way of bringing problems into more intense focus, primarily by identifying and defining goals in operational, action-oriented terms.

The systems approach can be regarded as a disciplined way of using knowledge from a variety of fields to analyze as precisely as possible sets of activities whose interrelationships are very complicated, and of formulating decision-relevant conclusions on the basis of that analysis. Since the systems way of thinking draws knowledge from a variety of disciplines and employs the technologies of many fields, it seems reasonable to assume that the systems approach is not a set, established process with clear-cut rules to follow in dealing with all problems (Pfeiffer, 1968). In other words, we may discover that there are several systems approaches to a problem.

But, there does seem to be one overriding concern of systems thinking, that is, efficiency of operation or, put another way, the objective of reducing costs. A major function of the systems approach, then, is to reconcile objectives and costs. Two questions become paramount: (1) Is the objective meaningful, i.e., is it worthwhile or does it serve the public interest? And (2) is it "the one best way" to achieve the goal, i.e., are there alternative ways to achieve the same goals at less cost or more effectively at the same cost? Cost in this context means using up resources. It is usually measured in terms of dollars, but very often the real costs can be thought of in terms of time or physical resources.

Generally speaking, the systems approach begins by identifying what has to be done, which means specifying goals. This involves, as we have already said, defining goals in operational terms, in ways that identify specific, concrete actions. One strategy is to make goals explicit from objectives. A goal in this case becomes a general description of purpose or desired outcome which can be accomplished by meeting one or more objectives. Objectives on the other hand are defined as clear statements of measurable and/or intended results which identify the conditions and criteria under which the results will take place. Objectives imply or make explicit certain action steps and activities which must be accomplished by a specific time or in a specific sequence. A goal is not achieved by a single activity but is established with the intent that success is dependent upon several activities. We assume that if the goal is met, then a series of prior accomplishments (objectives) were fulfilled.

Once the goal statement is specified in terms of objectives, action steps, and activities, criteria are then selected which measure how well the objectives are being met and determine when those objectives have been reached.

Once objectives and criteria have been determined, the next step calls for identifying and spelling out different methods of meeting each objective. This process must be systematic, and it becomes the most creative phase of the systems approach. From the point of view of evaluation, this process demands knowledge about the service being offered, the delivery system within which the service is being offered, and some understanding of the value orientations of the funding group, the service providers and the recipients of services.

From the point of view of evaluation, while alternatives are generally evaluated in quantitative terms, qualitative factors need to be considered also. There are always political implications, questions of morale, and other effects which must be taken into account while judging the worth or effectiveness of a particular activity .

Summary. So far, what I have tried to point out is that the so-called "systems" part of the systems approach contributes to our technology of evaluative research in the following ways:

1. It provides us with a disciplined way of thinking in which one criterion

of effectiveness is the reconciliation of goals and resources. In other words, in terms of decision making, we cannot anticipate goal attainment if the resources are inadequate.

This is an important concept for us in the fields of human services planning because too often we begin with too little too late; in which case, we are destined to failure. We have witnessed this phenomenon time and time again. The war on poverty of the 1960s is a good example; Medicare for the elderly is another example.

2. The systems approach provides us with a logical framework within which to assess efficiency of operation. The technique which has become most popular is cost-benefit analysis.

3. The power of the systems approach lies fundamentally in the striking fact that it can promote and amplify incisive decision making. It requires a specific set of procedures in the goal-setting process (Pfeiffer, 1968).

The first task is *Defining the System's Objectives*—a basic problem in human services planning is the establishment of clear and precise objectives. Wholey et al. (1970) in their study of federal social programs found that in most programs, objectives were not established; output measures had not been selected; reporting systems did not yield information on the effects of programs or even on progress toward short-term objectives. They concluded: "The most clear-cut evidence of the primitive state of federal self-evaluation lies in the widespread failure of agencies even to spell out program objectives."

The second task of the goal-setting process is *Obtaining Measures of Effectiveness*—measuring the wrong things may be as unproductive as selecting the wrong objectives. Approximate yardsticks are therefore essential to goal setting, for making improvements on schedules and for keeping tabs on how closely the schedules are being met.

Once measures of effectiveness have been identified, the next task of the systems analyst is to *Identify Constraints and Uncontrollable Variables*—since every system is a part of a larger system, there will always be things that do not change and cannot be changed in any reasonable length of time. These are known as constraints and range from fixed budgets and existing rules and laws to firmly established traditions, special interest groups and coalitions, governmental structures, and political ethos. They must be considered because they have a profound effect on the capacity of a program to mount efficient and effective services.

The final task in the goal-setting process is the *Identification of Controllable Variables*—the systems approach views controllable variables as resources. As opposed to constraints, which are viewed as lying outside the system and over which the system has no control, resources are viewed as being within the system. They are the means that the system uses to do its job. Typically, when we turn to the measurement of resources, we do so in terms of money, of man hours, and of equipment. Resources, as opposed to constraints, are the things the system can change and use to its own advantage.

Having provided some framework within which to link the systems approach to evaluation, let's turn our attention briefly to the underlying concepts of evaluation.

Program Evaluation

Evaluation is defined as the process of determining the value or amount of success a particular intervention has had in terms of costs and benefits and goal attainment. It is also concerned with assessing the relevance (significance) and appropriateness of the stated goal, the feasibility of attaining it, as well as the value or impact of unintended outcomes.

This conception of evaluation is used because it emphasizes the relationship between evaluation and decision making, particularly decisions concerning the continuation, modification, expansion, or elimination of programs. In using program evaluation in this fashion the decision maker needs to determine, first, whether or not the program was carried out in accordance with the prescriptions set forth in the planning and development stages and, second, whether or not it worked. He also tries to ascertain whether the expenditure of resources has been efficient in comparison with alternative means of achieving the same objective.

Evaluation should be considered an integral part of a management process and therefore provide decision-relevant data in four categories: (1) compliance control, (2) performance, (3) efficiency, and (4) accountability.

Compliance Control. The evaluator collects data about whether the program is carried out in accordance with the prescriptions set forth in the planning and development stage. Some people refer to this as program monitoring.

Program monitoring may be distinguished from evaluation in that it rarely questions the relevance or the rationale of the program. It begins with a predetermined model which describes how the program should be administered. It is usually conducted on an ongoing basis while the program is still in operation. It seeks to respond to questions about the extent to which procedures and practices need to be modified in order to conform to an original plan or to operate more efficiently. It involves on-site visits and focuses upon whether the staff measures up to predetermined qualifications. It seeks to determine if the administrative hierarchy and table of organization as planned are operative, if proper reporting forms and procedures are being used as planned, and whether services are being provided as originally conceived.

It should be remembered that while on-site monitoring can generally be implemented immediately, it is sometimes difficult to develop objective standards to use in assessing program operations. To minimize subjectivity, strategies of compliance control should be structured around performance evaluations.

Performance. Decision questions relative to performance seek to determine whether the program worked. They provide data from which the administrator can make judgments about continuation, modification, expansion, or elimination of programs or program components.

Performance evaluation (sometimes referred to as plan versus performance evaluation) is carried out by comparing the plan with actual performance. Comparisons are made on input, process, and output measures.

This evaluation strategy requires data about the recipient of services, service delivery structure, process flow, component success as well as overall program effectiveness. Much of these data should be built into the organization's planning and control system which provides the structure through which data flow into the evaluation system and results flow out to support administrative decisions.

The performance criterion addresses issues concerned with the extent to which the program serves empirically established needs and whether program goals imply need reduction, and the extent to which goals serve the public interest. The concept *empirically established needs* refers to a systematic codification of needs within the target population. This process may involve the use of some form of survey research by which needs assessment is conducted or it may be some organized method for identifying unmet needs. The term *public interest* carries a distributive connotation and refers to benefits to society. In its most general use it refers to the well-being of every member of society. The heart of program evaluation is the measurement of change. Change, then, is defined as progress in the direction of society's ideals. It can be assumed that the social welfare function (public interest) of human services programs is change—which leads to social equity and social opportunity. Indicators of program performance are measures of the extent to which program activities have led to mastery over one's environment or the acquisition of new coping skills.

Efficiency. The evaluator collects data about whether expenditures of resources have been efficient in comparison with alternative means of achieving the same goal. Assessing program efficiency is related to measuring how economically the program accomplishes its goal. It is concerned with two questions: (1) what is the extent of waste, duplication, and inefficiency, and (2) are there alternative programs which can achieve the same goals at less cost or more effectively at the same cost? As already stated, questions of efficiency usually involve cost-benefit analysis.

The efficiency criterion is usually applied when there is need to make some changes in the allocation of resources. This may include changes in:

+ The amount allocated
+ The combinations of resources allocated
+ The purposes for which resources are allocated
+ The timetables for allocation
+ Procedures of allocation
+ The criteria for allocation

Accountability. Accountability evolves from a relationship in which someone or group in authority delegates to another the responsibility for providing certain services in exchange for certain compensation, benefits, or incentives.

For most human services organizations, authority rests in some legislative body, legislative mandate, or governing group. Accountability assumes the existence of an agreement that the authority has been designated and accepted by one party to perform certain activities on behalf of another. It assumes consensus as to the criteria by which performance will be measured and expectations are stated in the form of some contract or compact.

Human services programs are accountable both to the authority under whose auspices the programs operate and the recipients of the services.

As depicted in Figure 1, human services programs can be viewed as a system with three component parts: (1) the donor subsystem, (2) the service delivery subsystem, and (3) the recipient subsystem. The service delivery subsystem intersects with the donor subsystem at Interface 1 and with the recipient subsystem at Interface 2. The task of the evaluator, then, is to measure the quality of the two interfaces.[2]

The measure of Interface 1 is a measure of compliance. The primary question to be answered is: Is the program doing what it said it would do? The measure of Interface 2 is a determination of the extent to which the service provider affords the recipient opportunity to gain mastery over his environment or improved life chances. Questions to be answered by the evaluator include:

1. Does the program provide the recipient with a viable course of redress?

2. Is the recipient able to influence decisions that affect his circumstances?

Figure 1. Relationship of Intra-System Components

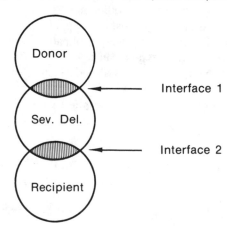

3. To what extent are decision makers (donor subsystem) responsive and sensitive to recipient needs and interests?

Inferring from Figure 1, then, measures of accountability are defined in terms of compliance and responsiveness to consumer needs. Compliance control has already been discussed. Responsiveness to consumer needs relates to the *availability* of services and the *efficiency* in the delivery of services. Kaplan et al. (1972) suggested that the availability of service can be examined from two dimensions: (1) accessibility—the ease with which the consumer is able to enter the system, and (2) continuity—the ease with which the consumer is able to move within the system. Efficiency in the delivery of services is measured in terms of reduction of costs and of duplication of service delivery, and in terms of economies of scale.

In short, evaluation can be viewed as a judgment of worth and a process for measuring the degree to which the real world matches the judgment of what is desired. An evaluation should not be undertaken unless there is a clear understanding of the decisions to be supported by that evaluation, and should not only measure goal attainment, compliance, performance, and efficiency, but it should also seriously question the premise on which the program is based.

Now that we have established some general parameters for conducting program evaluation, let's turn to the primary objective of this paper—that is, to link the systems approach to program evaluation.

Systems Approach to Program Evaluation

A systems approach to program evaluation begins from the premise that the evaluator must assess the performance of the *total system*. As a model of evaluation, the systems approach to evaluation differs from other analytical models in that, as we said earlier, the systems approach is essentially *deductive* rather than *inductive*. This is an important distinction because the inductive method is associated more frequently with the scientific method, and its concern is with establishing empirical relationships between cause and effect. The systems approach is less concerned with cause-effect relationships than it is with the maximum performance of the total operation and the interdependent relationships of the component parts.

The systems model is concerned principally with efficiency and the reduction of costs in providing services and relates primarily to questions of resource allocations. It assumes that certain resources must be devoted to essential nongoal activities such as maintenance and preservation of the system. From this viewpoint, the central question in an evaluation of the effectiveness of an intervention should be: How close does the organization's allocation of resources approach an optimum distribution? Etzioni (1969), a central proponent of this model, suggests that what really is important is whether there exists a balanced distribution of resources among all organizational needs rather than the maximal satisfaction of any single organizational requirement.

The systems model of evaluation assumes that the evaluator must answer at least four questions: (1) How effective is the coordination of organizational subunits? (2) How adequate are the resources? (3) How adaptive is the organization to environmental and internal demands? (4) Were the goals and subgoals met?

While the measurement of general organizational goals are central to the systems model, proponents of the systems model tend to minimize the need to measure how well a *specific* organizational goal is achieved. They contend that such a strategy is unproductive and often misleading since an organization constantly functions at a variety of levels with a variety of goals which are sometimes conflicting. Moreover, they contend, overattention to a specific goal will lead to underconcern for other programmatic functions. The fact that an organization can become less effective by allocating excessive means to achieve a particular goal is viewed by systems protagonists as just as detrimental as withholding such resources.

The systems model of evaluation tends to be more productive in decision making among organizations which employ program budgeting. The general idea of program budgeting is that budgetary decisions should be made by focusing upon overall goals. In other words, program budgeting is a goal-oriented program structure which presents data on all of the operations and activities of the program in categories which reflect the program's goals. Inputs, such as personnel, equipment, and maintenance are considered only in relationship to program outcomes. Program budgeting then lays heavy emphasis upon relating costs to accomplishing the overall goal.

Management Information Systems. The typical strategy of systems evaluation is the assessment of input, process, and output activities. This generally requires an elaborate planning and control system through which flow data for evaluation and out of which flows information to support administrative decisions. This system is typically called a Management Information System (MIS).

A carefully planned MIS also incorporates the concept of a total system and working downward through all the subsystems. In other words, an effective MIS looks down from the top, the natural vantage point of the decision makers who will use it. An MIS should be designed so as to focus on the critical tasks and decisions made within the organization and to provide the kind of information that the decision maker needs to perform those tasks and make those decisions (Zani, 1970). To facilitate evaluation, the MIS must incorporate 11 essential data elements.

1. Needs—areas of perceived void or lack of services
2. Goals—general statements revealing assumptions made about expected outcomes of an organized program. Goals identify a program area, its target, purpose, and expected results.

3. Objectives—specific statements written in measurable terms which describe a target population, treatment to be given, results expected, expected completion dates, and specific individuals who will accomplish the tasks

4. Resources—the human, technological, and organizational materials available for use in meeting goals and objectives

5. Constraints—factors which limit the scope and feasibility of objectives (e.g., lack of funds, limited supply of trained personnel)

6. Strategies—the "plans for action," the methods or procedures for determining what activities will be used

7. Selection criteria—bases for the selection of the particular activities or operations

8. Choice—selection of operational strategy or plan of action

9. Implementation—initial operationalization of strategy or putting the operational plan to work

10. Evaluation—delineating, obtaining, and providing useful information for making decisions concerning the program components or results of activities

11. Feedback—information from evaluation which has implications for future activities or planning (Stedman and Surles, 1972)

Steps in "Systems" Evaluation. Once the organization has developed an adequate information and reporting system, program evaluation is relatively straightforward. As indicated earlier, the logical framework of the systems approach is:

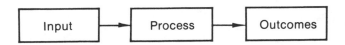

Expressed in terms of a set of linked evaluation hypotheses, the evaluation strategy presumes:

1. If *inputs*, then *process*
2. If *process*, then *outcomes*
3. If *outcomes*, then *purpose*
4. If *purpose*, then *goal attainment*

I. Measuring quality of inputs: The first step is to assess the quality of inputs. This involves the evaluation of:

    A. Organizational competence

        1. Organizational practices and activities

            a. *Conflict and inconsistency*—the degree to which policies, procedures, standards of performance, and directions are inconsistent or inconsistently applied, e.g., program objectives are inconsistent

b. *Formalization*—the degree to which standard practices, policies, and position responsibilities are explicitly formalized, e.g., written procedures are available

c. *Job pressure*—the degree to which there is adequate time and manpower to accomplish tasks, e.g., too much or too little to do

d. *Work flow coordination*—the degree to which staffing patterns and job responsibilities are coordinated

2. Decision making and communication structure

a. *Goal consensus and clarity*—the nature of organizational objectives and degree to which objectives are clear and agreed upon by staff

b. *Planning adequacy*—the degree to which organizational objectives are viewed as adequate to accomplish organizational goals

c. *Adequacy of authority*—the degree to which staff perceive that authority is delegated consistently with job demands, e.g., "I have enough authority to handle problems"

d. *Communication processes*—the availability or completeness of communication flow; the amount of perceived information distortion and suppression; the nature of upward information reporting requirements

3. Identification with the organization

a. *Role conflict*—the degree of incongruency or incompatibility in the performance requirements of individual roles

b. *Role ambiguity*—the predictability of the outcome or responses to behavior; the existence or clarity of behavioral requirements which would serve to guide behavior and provide knowledge that the behavior is appropriate

c. *Motivational characteristics*—the degree of psychological participation in terms of influence in job activities, decision making, idea transmittal, degree of task autonomy, degree of intrinsic motivation

d. *Work alienation*—satisfaction with present job as based on original job expectation

B. Client inputs

1. Are services directed at the appropriate client group?

2. Is the size of the client group large enough to justify the resources required?

This phase of the evaluation relies heavily upon questionnaires, attitude scales, checklists, in-depth interviews, and site visitations. Data from this phase of the evaluation are frequently referred to as "soft data" in that they are derived principally from qualitative methodology.

II. Measuring organizational process: The second step in the systems approach to program evaluation is to assess modes of client processing. This aspect of the evaluation focuses upon the client pathway from entry to exit, and usually begins with a "mapping" of a client through the system. During this procedure the evaluator looks for factors which facilitate or limit the following:

A. Availability of services—the extent to which services respond to empirically established needs

B. Accessibility of services—the ease with which the consumer is able to enter the system

C. Continuity of services—the ease with which the consumer is able to move within the system at different points in time. The evaluator is also concerned with lateral coordination among service units, improved planning, improved efficiency in resource use, and improved communication in relationship to policy making, program design, and implementation.

This phase of the evaluation also employs qualitative methodology. Its strengths lie in the expertise of the evaluator as well as in its procedures for "getting close to the data." Data analysis is not wholly qualitative, however. Sometimes the data so observed and collected are used in the development of scales for rating and scoring, and for comparing individuals and groups. At times, data may be subjected to other statistical procedures to determine the extent to which two or more kinds of observations made on an individual or group have a tendency to be related or found together (correlation), or to determine the extent to which one or several observed items may be causally related to another and therefore usable to predict the other (causal analysis).

III. Measuring organizational outcomes: Measuring program results is the heart of most evaluation efforts. The systems approach, because of its emphasis upon efficiency, relies primarily upon cost-benefit analysis for outcome evaluation.

Cost-benefit analysis is a technique which concerns itself with the optimum allocation of resources. It is a tool of analysis which assesses alternative courses of action in order to help decision makers to maximize the net benefit to society. The essence of this analysis lies in its ability to evaluate the total value of benefits against the total costs.

Second, it is often desirable that the list of benefits and costs, both private or social, be expressed as monetary values in order to arrive at an estimate of the current net benefits of a program. The benefits and costs are usually reflected via the price mechanism through the working of the market forces of supply and demand. In certain circumstances, however, market forces may fail to reflect all costs and benefits. This is the fundamental distinction between private and social costs and benefits. Therefore, the quantification of all costs and benefits of a program is difficult, if not at times virtually impossible. Assuming that these difficulties have been surmounted, the analyst is left with an estimate of net benefits of the project.

Finally, a comparison must be made of the stream of annual net benefits and the cost stream of the program. There are three basic alternative criteria in evaluating a program: the benefit-cost ratio, the internal rate of return, or the present value of net benefits. Each criterion has its own advantages and the evaluator must be clear about how he is going to use the data in order to determine which is most appropriate. Since each requires a different set of assumptions and different procedures, their results may not be consistent with each other.

In any case, however, in order to apply these criteria, cost-benefit analysis has to make assumptions as to the size of the rate of interest which is to reflect the social or private opportunity cost rate of investment funds. Unfortunately, there are many rates of interest observed in the market, each reflecting the yield on alternative types and mixes of investments.

Since the choice of a specific discount factor is so highly speculative and since computers are available to many evaluators, it is very informative to compute cost-benefit data for several discount rates.

The cost-benefit calculus is not a wholly satisfactory tool for evaluating human services programs, because of its incapability to measure "psychic" or "social" benefits. Psychic and social benefits are defined here to refer to the state or well-being of the recipient or the changes that take place in attitude and behavior as outcomes. Weisbrod (1969) argues that an evaluation design built around cost-benefit analysis is likely to reach negative conclusions about the effectiveness of any human services program since only "economic" benefits and costs are taken into account. (Remember, an evaluation design built upon the systems approach is concerned primarily with "allocative efficiency.")

One of the precautions in interpreting cost-benefit data relates to the fact that, while a particular human services program may be judged inefficient, it may not necessarily be considered undesirable. It may, for example, have certain favorable income redistribution consequences that are socially preferable to other benefits.

There is general agreement that the utility of a cost-benefit model as an evaluative tool lies in its emphasis on a systematic examination of alternative courses of action and their implications. But it is important to note that data from such a model should be only one piece of evidence in the appraisal process; and, from the vantage point of the evaluator who is concerned more with "social" than economic benefits, such data may not be the most significant piece of evidence. When programs have goals that go beyond simply maximizing the return on public investments irrespective of who receives the benefits, a simple cost-benefit ratio is an insufficient indicator of program effectiveness.

Conclusion

This paper set out to present a systems approach to program evaluation. It began from the premise that the systems perspective offers program administrators a framework within which to look first at the total organization and then the interrelationship of component parts, meshing simultaneously toward circumscribed goals.

The characteristics of the systems approach is that it is deductive in character and emphasizes efficiency of operation. To achieve efficiency of operation, the model presumes that there must exist a balanced distribution of resources among all organizational units. Therefore, an evaluation strategy must include measures of input, process, and outcome variables.

A major contribution of the systems approach to program evaluation is the systematic process by which the evaluator arrives at judgments about the effectiveness of program inputs. While the model does not place as much emphasis upon measuring goal attainment as other models, it does nonetheless offer a logical framework for goal setting and selecting alternative strategies for goal attainment.

The systems approach to program evaluation relies heavily upon systems analysis for measuring outcomes. Systems analysis is a quantitative analysis and is concerned principally with the assessment of costs and benefits. Therefore, cost-benefit analysis is the primary evaluative tool.

The weakness of the systems approach to program evaluation is the inherent weakness of the cost-benefit calculus to measure certain social benefits of social interventions. Many programs are desirable, and therefore effective, not because they are cost-beneficial, but rather because they serve the public interest and are, therefore, worthwhile.

Notes

1. General systems theory seeks to classify systems by the way their components are organized (interrelated) and to derive the "laws," or typical patterns of behavior, for the different classes of systems singled out by the taxonomy. Cybernetics is the science of communication and control. It examines patterns of signals by means of which information is transmitted within a system and from one system to another. Transmission of information is essential in control, and the capacity of a system to exercise control depends on how much information it can process and store. A central concept of cybernetics is "quantity of information" which relates to the number of "decisions" which must be made in order to reduce the range of possible answers to the question one asks; to put it another way, to reduce uncertainty.

Information theory (also called communication theory) has to do with the abstract logical nature of information, its mathematical measure, and the notions of structure, organization, control, order, and entropy. From these concepts come the notion of a decision-making system (a device for processing, storing, and retrieving information), and the concept that information can be processed only if the decisions (that is, events within the organism conditional upon other events) are integrated and meshed in certain ways (Buckley, 1968).

2. This concept was originally developed by Leonard Goodwin in "On

making research relevant to social policy and national problem solving," *American Psychologist*, 26 (5), May 1971.

References

Buckley, W. *Modern systems research for the behavioral scientist*. Chicago: Aldine Publishing Co., 1968.

Churchman, D. W. *The systems approach*. New York: Dell Publishing Co., 1968.

Etzioni, A. Two approaches to organizational analysis: A critique and a suggestion. In Herbert C. Schulberg, et al., *Program evaluation in the health fields*. New York: Behavioral Publications, 1969.

Kaplan, J., et al. Planning—facilities, programs, and services—government and nongovernment. *Gerontologist*, 12 (2), 1972, 36–48.

Pfeiffer, J. *A new look at education: Systems analysis in our schools and colleges*. New York: The Odyssey Press, 1968.

Stedman, D. J., and Surles, R. C. Essentials of program evaluation. In *Synergism for the seventies*. Reston, Va.: Council for Exceptional Children, 1972.

Washington, R. O. *Program evaluation in the human services*. Milwaukee, Wisconsin: Center for Advanced Studies in Human Services, University of Wisconsin, 1975.

Weisbrod, B. A. Benefits of manpower programs. Theoretical and methodological issues. In G. G. Somens and W. D. Wood (Eds.), *Cost-benefit analysis of manpower policies*. Ontario: Queens University, 1969.

Wholey, J. S., et al. *Federal evaluation policy: Analyzing the effects of public programs*. Urban Institute, 1970.

Zani, William. Blueprint for MIS. *Harvard Business Review*, Nov.–Dec. 1970, 95–100.

Basic Course Design in Gerontology: Overview and Issues

Ruth B. Weg
University of Southern California

Design has many meanings: intention, purpose, end, to plan the form and structure, to intend for a definite purpose, and adaptation of means to a preconceived end (all from the *Random House Dictionary*, 1967). The charge to this group is to explore the development of those courses which are considered fundamental to gerontology.

There are multidimensional aspects to designing a program for learning gerontology. We need to know what we are designing, for whom, and at which specific level. Course design relates to the how, to content, and to form. Other concerns in planning courses include design for now, for the future; design for work and design for change.

What, Who

The design for learning relates to attitudes, skills, and knowledge necessary for the varied personnel involved in the expanding programs in aging within the educational enterprise (both in number and depth) and in programs for and with older persons. That personnel ranges from those in doctoral and postdoctoral study who conceivably represent the cadre of leadership among the researchers, teachers, top-level planners, and administrators to those who work on a one-to-one basis with older persons. But the greatest need of all parallels the enormous increase in programs and activities directly for and with the elders: community and day care centers, convalescent and nursing homes, residential communities, community college programs, counseling, legal services, and protective services. It is this group of people who need be not only exposed, but immersed in the facts, the potential, and effect in the field. They become knowledgeable in the doing, in the real world of hierarchies, red tape, difficult people, situations, and opportunities.

The design for learning in gerontology also involves educational opportunities for older persons seeking continued involvement or reacquaintance with sources of information that will contribute to those coping capacities necessary for the fast change artist that is contemporary culture.

The education of those in existing professions whose work touches older persons—physicians, nurses, pharmacists, psychologists, hospital and nursing home administrators, occupational and physical therapists, and dental hygienists—is central to the present requirements of gerontology as a scholarly inquiry and the significant application of its findings in practice. Many have called this education and/or training "gerontologizing" the professions.

And finally, the overall design for education in gerontology relates to the enlightenment of the "everyman and everywoman" student. They can look forward to their adult development without fear and ignorance as they and the society in which they live change attitudes toward the later years of life. In view of the current and anticipated numbers of older people in our society, it makes good sense that all students experience consciousness raising about the life span continuum and the meaning of aging within it.

Aging Content and Effect

Aging is hardly a single process or concept, related only to physiology, or psyche, or to sociological and environmental factors. Rather, aging is most readily explored by examining the interactions among all aspects in human growth and function. One can construct a fairly basic course as an overview, multidisciplinary and issue oriented. This kind of introductory course can be used as general education for the everyman and everywoman student or as an open door into gerontology for those who become committed to the study of aging and/or older persons.

The necessity for basic courses is clear. The content and form of these courses can and does take many shapes. Any one basic course may concentrate in psychological, physiological, or sociological dimensions of aging. There are basic courses in ethnicity and aging, in aging and the environment, in tasks of the life cycle. Potential exists for course development in any and all aspects of human development and its interaction with a social, physical, and personal environment.

Too frequently however, the integration of each discipline's facts and figures with any of the others is lost. The specific content may remain unconnected to the wider view of human existence. Implications for the overall human condition is ignored. Further, these courses often omit the important undergirding for student capacity to function into the future, and may neglect to nourish sensitivity to the changing perspectives in gerontology. For those students who expect to be the practitioners in gerontology, this sensitivity is especially important for a future which will undoubtedly present new challenges.

The levels of the student populations will determine the emphases and directions of the courses. These may be quite different for the paraprofessional, lay audiences, baccalaureate students, those in a discrete gerontology program, those in the liberal arts, the master's level, both within a particular discipline and in gerontology, certificate-seeking students, the requirements of the doctoral and postdoctoral levels, the continuing education of those at work in the field, older persons, and those professionals described earlier.

A Sequence in Course Building

It is necessary to gather, evaluate, and coordinate available gerontological information before designing a course. There is information available organized along disciplinary, interdisciplinary, and multidisciplinary lines and at different levels of sophistication. Further, worthwhile materials can be found not only in the plethora of texts that seem to be tumbling out at a phenomenal pace—but in the increasing number of journals that report and comment on the research and practices in aging. There are now proceedings of symposia, seminars, and volumes containing the thinking and the works of many competent colleagues, dealing with theoretical and practical issues.

Course(s) and curriculum design take into consideration the many aspects of the particular student population, informational needs, past educational levels, and career goals. In addition to factual, theoretical materials, a number of courses need to move beyond the traditional text and lectures, and demonstrate concern with experiential input, with audiovisual and community resources, in persons and settings for field experiences.

It is helpful to develop an estimate of faculty and graduate student talent and interest so that any course, or sequence of courses will be mounted in the most attractive, effective way within a particular institutional setting. Energy and expertise may be in a department, a program, an institute, or a center. It can be possible to invite this collegial expertise as a contribution from neighboring departments or disciplines. On the other hand, it may be necessary to buy the time of a faculty member.

In order for gerontology to continue to grow into a coherent, healthy academic structure, a course(s) must be consistent with other courses or programs more indirectly related to gerontology. There is no particular virtue in the overelaboration of courses. Philosophical concepts and operational details require discussion among the responsible, involved faculty and administrative staff. A necessary step is the construction of logical course sequences in terms of objectives and methodology for each course, and the gerontological curriculum as a whole. Each level of information becomes more meaningful if it articulates well with other levels, and ultimately with the real world of aging outside the educational institution.

Finally, as with any educational program, an essential part of planning integrates mechanisms for evaluation and change. In order to determine the effectiveness and appropriateness of any course design, early identification of criteria, objectives, methodologies for presentation, and modes of evaluation ensures more logical structure organically relating these parameters to the content design.

The Educated Person in Gerontology:
The Danger of Vocational Training

Let us look at the characteristics of the educated person in gerontology. My own present concern with this notion stems from the resurgence of "training" for a particular job—a moment in time—the "vocational" cry. It is understandable in these days of inflation and serious unemployment, that today's student looks to specific education which best prepares for available work. However, the capitulation of education to narrow vocationalism may indeed be a disservice to real understanding and employability of the job seeker. Postindustrial society makes no promise of "this is your job and/or career" into perpetuity. The movement of events is at streak speed—and tomorrow is almost always here. In my opinion, nothing can more severely damage the growth of gerontology and the future careers therein so much as the arteriosclerotic effect of vocational training. Professional/practitioner education of the late twentieth and twenty-first centuries cannot afford the luxury of these limiting educational objectives.

The educated person in gerontology is not only the revered researcher and/or theoretician who provides the lifeline of new knowledge to teachers, practitioners, older persons, and the community at large—is not only the practitioner on the "firing line" in programs with and for older persons—is not only the "teacher" who will transmit to a variety of students, media, and publics, but may indeed be shades and combinations of all three, permutations that develop quite naturally in different situations.

The educated person in gerontology has learned to listen well, to think critically about the printed and oral message, has the ability to use information however the knowledge is explored, and has a grasp of the significant overall concepts and issues in aging that remain useful for individuals and society in face of rapid, ephemeral change.

The Opportunity

It is with curriculum building in this most recent, academic multidiscipline, gerontology, that opportunity presents itself to avoid some obvious difficulties in "typical" basic courses. It is possible to use only that portion of traditional methodology, the "tried and true" presentations and requirements, that really works in terms of stated objectives and outcomes. Students and faculty alike could stretch their thinking by the combination of the nontraditional, the untried with the best of tradition. In a field yet unfettered by academic ritual, let us not imitate in the hope of approval and status—both more satisfactorily achieved with original, creative, yet realistic approaches.

Basic courses in the many-leveled, multipurpose programs play a primary role. Such courses lay the knowledge base essential to dispel the widely held, mistaken images of aging and older persons, fed largely on ignorance. Since there is at least a minimum body of knowledge appropriate to all who would learn about aging, commonalities exist in the "basic courses" wherever they may be found. The basic concepts and issues are shared among all curricula at whatever level.

It is in the attempt to meet the unique requirements of each gerontological structure (student body, faculty, programmatic and career objectives) that the creative differences will be apparent. All have the same long-range focus—to so alter the informational level and consequent behavior of individuals and society at large that the functional reality of gerontology and older persons will move forward. The balance in structure and content of courses in gerontology, will hopefully represent the net effect of many processes in an overall creative undertaking.

A closing note that reflects the continual tension inherent in intellectual and academic growth seems appropriate in this search for logical development in gerontology.

> *Tradition itself cannot constitute a creative force. It always has a decadent tendency to promote formalization and repetition. What is needed to direct it into creative channels is a fresh energy which repudiates dead forms and prevents living ones from becoming static. In one sense, for a tradition to live, it must constantly be destroyed. At the same time, destruction by itself clearly cannot create new cultural forms. There must be some other force which restrains destructive energy and prevents it from reducing all about it to havoc. The dialectical synthesis of tradition and antitradition is the structure of true creativeness.*[1]

Note

1. Tange Kenzo, "Katsura—Tradition and Creation in Japanese Architecture," in S. Gould (Chairman, Commission on Nontraditional Study), *Diversity by Design* (San Francisco: Jossey-Bass, 1973), p. 1.